Karen Minden

BAMBOO STONE
The Evolution of a Chinese Medical Elite

BAMBOO STONE

Cleaving to the mountain never letting go
Roots sunk deeply in jagged stone
Still standing strong and firm after many storms
No matter what direction the wind blows.

by Zheng Banqiao, Qing dynasty poet

竹石

鄭燮　板橋

咬定青山不放鬆

立根原在破岩中

千磨萬擊還堅勁

任爾東西南北風

BAMBOO STONE

The Evolution of
a Chinese
Medical Elite

Karen Minden

UNIVERSITY OF TORONTO PRESS
Toronto Buffalo London

© University of Toronto Press Incorporated 1994
Toronto Buffalo London
Printed in Canada

ISBN 0–8020–0550–0

Printed on acid-free paper

Canadian Cataloguing in Publication Data

Minden, Karen, 1949–
Bamboo stone: the evolution of
a Chinese medical elite
Includes bibliographical references and index.
ISBN 0-8020-0550-0
1. Medical education – China – History – 20th century.
2. Physicians – China. 3. Missionaries, Medical – China.
4. Missionaries, Medical – Canada.
5. Hua hsi ta hsueh. College of Medicine and Dentistry.
6. Hua hsi ta hsueh. College of Medicine and Dentistry – Alumni.
I. Title.
R602.M55 1994   610'.951   C94-930018-7

University of Toronto Press acknowledges the
financial assistance to its publishing program
of the Canada Council and the
Ontario Arts Council.

This book has been published
with the help of a grant from the
Social Science Federation of Canada,
using funds provided by the
Social Sciences and Humanities Research Council of Canada.

Contents

Maps, Figure, Tables

Maps

Figure

Tables

Preface

The internationalization of higher education has been an increasing trend for almost a century, as students from developing economies seek Western education in the sciences as a key to economic prosperity. The implications for the resulting cross-fertilization of ideas, technology, and culture have become a topic of interest to scholars of economic development, political modernization, and scientific advancement. The 'reverse brain drain' experienced by South Korea and Taiwan in the 1980s, a phenomenon that will contribute to bridging the cultural and economic gap between Asia and the West, is only the most recent manifestation of a process that has seen the emergence of a Western-trained intellectual and technological elite in the developing world. The aim of this book is to elucidate the process and long-term implications of technology transfer through higher education. It is hoped that it will be useful to policy-makers, development specialists, China scholars, and those interested in cross-cultural relations in education, trade, and development assistance.

A Note about Romanization

The *pinyin* system of romanization of Chinese names and words has been used in this text. The exceptions occur where there is no written record of a name in Chinese characters, and therefore the exact pronunciation is unknown. Since the *pinyin* system was not introduced in China until after 1949, the archival records use various spellings for Chinese names. Where there is a clear equivalent in *pinyin*, this has been used. When there is uncertainty about the correct pronunciation, the archival form has been retained. In cases of well-known names, the original spelling appears in parentheses. The only exception is the name *Chiang Kai-shek*, whose Mandarin name, *Jiang Jie-shi*, is not in common usage.

Acknowledgments

This was a project about people, and there are many who gave their time and assistance in guiding me through the past and present in both China and Canada. Many years ago, Professor B. Michael Frolic pointed a very sceptical graduate student towards the United Church of Canada Archives in Toronto. The research became a fascinating journey through time and between cultures, and I thank my teachers at York University, University of Toronto, and University of California at Berkeley for contributing to my knowledge and understanding of China. I am indebted to Jerome Chen, Victor Falkenheim, AnElissa Lucas, Mary Bullock, and Ruth Hayhoe for the intellectual inspiration of their ideas in the early stages of the research. In addition to her own scholarship, which allowed me to develop some of my ideas, Ruth Hayhoe provided encouragement and support. Arthur Waldron provided the impetus to persist and also the vital links with scholars in China who were interested in the historical implications of Western education for China's development. Beth Goldstein, Oscar Marantz, Zhang Guo-liang, and Xiao Hong provided invaluable assistance in the design and evaluation of the research survey; Ward Struthers provided expert technical assistance in analysing survey data.

The missionaries and alumni of West China Union University who responded to my questions were unstinting in their generosity during the years of research. In Canada, Mr William Small, Ms Evelyn Ricker, and Professor Stephen Endicott

made it possible for me to contact the missionaries who had
served in West China. Dr Gordon Campbell, the late Drs
Ralph Outerbridge and Frederick Kao showed constant enthusiasm and provided wise counsel. Dr Peggy Falkenheim and Ms
Jan Dick each contributed to the success of my efforts to carry
out research in Chengdu. In China, Dr Cao Zhongliang and Dr
Cao Zeyi made it possible for me to do the research for this
book. They and Dr George Deng, Dr Chen Zheng-yu, and the
faculty and staff of the International Office of West China
University of Medical Sciences always responded to my end-
less requests and provided warm hospitality during my visits
to the campus. Dr Stephan Yang was a beacon of light in the
early days of my research, helping me to plan and carry out
my task. In Beijing, Dr Tommy Hu arranged for me to meet
alumni and provided advice and friendship. Mrs Esther Huang
and Dr Denny Huang opened their home to me in Hong Kong
and arranged for interviews with alumni. In Chengdu, I was
greatly assisted in archival research and evaluation of information by patient and knowledgable professors, including Drs
C.C. Chen, Franklin Wu, Liu Zheng-gang, Peng Shu-yi, Zhu
Ling, and Bill Qiu and his student Kathleen. Professor Gu
Xuejia of Sichuan University was kind enough to share his
insights with me, and Mr Meng of the WCUMS Archives office
facilitated my research.

Financial support was generously provided by the Social
Sciences and Humanities Research Council of Canada,
through both a Private Scholars' Grant and, subsequently, a
Canada Research Fellowship. This provided me with the time
and resources to carry out a complex research agenda. My
sincere thanks are extended to the anonymous reviewers who
believed in the potential of this project. Support also came
from the York University–University of Toronto Joint Centre
for Asia Pacific Studies programme on Canadian missionaries
in East Asia, led by Peter Mitchell and Margo Gewurtz.

I am indebted to the staff of the United Church of Canada
Archives: Glenn Lucas, Neil Semple, Mary Ann Tyler, Mary
Tilley, Mark van Stempvoort, Rick Stapleton, and Gwen Nor-
man. The Tallin family were generous in allowing me access

to the family correspondence of Dr Gladys Cunningham. Omar Walmsley gave me the gift of his father's, Dr Lewis Walmsley's, book on the history of the West China Union University. Bertha Hensman provided the research material on the Kilborn family. The staff at the Rockefeller Archives Center in North Tarreytown, NY, and Drs Richard Howard and Chi Wang of the Library of Congress in Washington, DC, were most generous in their assistance. The Canadian Department of External Affairs allowed me access to its archives, and I am grateful to Ambassador Sidney Freifeld, Don Page, and Arthur Blanchette for their support.

Jane Curran and Oscar Marantz were thoughtful and diligent in their editing of the manuscript at its various stages. Linda Gransden and her staff were patient and untiring in preparing the manuscript.

I am fortunate to have made many friends in this endeavour. Each of the missionaries and alumni made me feel welcome and opened their hearts and minds to my probing questions. Dr George Deng guided me throughout, as mentor and friend. Although I am an outsider in both time and place with respect to the events described in this book, the alumni and missionaries made me feel a part of them.

I would like to express my sincere gratitude to Liu Guo Wu of Chengdu, who provided the calligraphy for the poem 'Bamboo Stone.' My thanks go also to Professor Richard King, who assisted with the translation. I am grateful to an anonymous Chinese physician who brought this poem to my attention.

My family in Toronto never failed to encourage and support this effort. They gave both intellectual and logistical support, and I am particularly grateful to my mother and father, who took over my parenting duties on many occasions, while I sequestered myself in archival research. My husband, Harvey Schipper, supported me as friend, colleague, and soundingboard, and was often left with the role of being father and mother over the years it took to complete this work. I am especially indebted to Harvey, and to our children, Rachel and Elyse, who made it take longer, but made it the more worthwhile.

I hope that my understanding of the events described in this book and their meaning is accurate. Any errors of interpretation or fact are my responsibility.

BAMBOO STONE
The Evolution of a Chinese Medical Elite

Introduction

In the early 1950s, professors of medicine at the Sichuan Medical College tore down the American wall charts illustrating blood cell morphology and replaced them with charts from the Soviet Union. This action was one more step in the radical transformation of China's intellectual structure under the guidance of the Soviet *laodage* (elder brothers).

The Sichuan Medical College was originally the medical and dental faculty of the West China Union University (WCUU), a joint venture by five Western mission boards.[1] In 1950, following the Soviet educational model of technical institutions, the various faculties at the university were disbanded and regrouped into professional training institutes.[2] The medical faculty took these changes in stride, realizing that the Communist regime would be imposing radical reforms that the professors had no power to resist. Perhaps these changes would be only superficial, an indication to the new ruling cadres that the professors would support the regime. In their own minds, they could continue to diagnose and solve problems as they had been trained to do by their foreign and foreign-trained teachers. For the Communists, however, the institutional changes marked the end of an era. To internalize the transformation, they embarked on a massive program to re-educate the intelligentsia – the bearers of ideas – to conform to the new regime.

This book looks at one group of the Chinese intelligentsia, the medical elite, to try to fathom the process of technology transfer over time and between cultures. Chapter 1 presents a framework in which to assess the cross-cultural transfer between Western medical missionaries and the Chinese medical elite whom they trained. It addresses the issues of foreigners in China and the role of a modernizing intellectual elite in Chinese society. Chapter 2 describes the context in which the medical missionaries introduced their ideas of medical care, medical education, and the organization of health care in early twentieth-century China. Chapter 3 introduces the missionaries, their goals, and their institutional model for transforming China's health care and, by extension, Chinese society. Chapter 4 focuses on the West China Union University and its College of Medicine and Dentistry, or *Hua Da*, as it was called in Chinese. The school was the institutional setting for the interaction of two cultures and for the transmission of the learning, technology, and organization of 'modern' Western medicine in West China. Chapter 5 explores the lives of the Chinese students who attended West China Union University by examining their socioeconomic background, motivations, and campus life over three generations spanning the end of the Qing dynasty through the Sino-Japanese War and, finally, the Civil War of 1945–9. Chapter 6 follows the career patterns of the alumni from 1949 to 1989. After the expulsion of the foreign missionaries in the early 1950s, the university was transformed and its faculty dispersed. The succeeding years saw the alumni, as China's medical elite, navigate the twists and turns of China's political development, as their role in medical modernization careened from foundation, to pariah, to foundation of a new order. Chapter 7 assesses the significance of the lives of these Western-trained scientists. By examining the nature of generational continuity, of the role of China's intellectual elite, and of the patterns of shifting educational models in China, it places the process of technology transfer over time and between cultures in a specific framework.

To approach a Sinocentric perspective of the meeting of East and West, the book traces the development of a Canadian missionary medical school in Chengdu from the turn of the century to 1952, interweaving the missionary experience with that of the Chinese students who sought Western learning, and then examining the careers of the Chinese graduates based on material gathered in dusty archives in Toronto, New York, Ottawa, and Chengdu, and on intensive interviews throughout China and in North America, culminating in the spring of 1989.

A distinguished Chinese professor of sociology, commenting on this foreign scholar's attempt to understand the training of Chinese at a Christian university over a sixty-year span, made the following comment: 'We have a saying in Chinese for what you are doing – *ge xie sao yang* – scratching an itch with high boots on.' A number of cross-cultural experiences in the course of this research have taught me that entering this study with a preconceived model was folly. When I organized the list of Chinese alumni by geographic location, it was returned to me in chronological order by 'generations.' When I portrayed the missionaries as culturally insensitive, I was chastised by their Chinese students, many of them well into their seventies, for misunderstanding the mutual devotion of many of the missionary educators and their students. When I surmised that the Chinese alumni were motivated by a fervent nationalism, I was gently corrected with the observation that *ai guo*, love of country, was not to be confused with the negative exclusiveness of national sentiment.

This sojourn into a rich archival record, and the witness of almost a hundred alumni and their missionary professors, was a journey into their minds to examine the perceptions of their lives, of their university, their teachers, and their students, of China and the West, of war and revolution, and of medicine. To the extent it was possible, I tried to shed my own conceptual baggage to sense what it felt like to be a young missionary sailing from Vancouver for the remote vastness of West China. What was it like for the young and eager Chinese students to leave their Confucian family courtyard for the crowded dormitory of a Christian university? And most important, what ideas did the graduates carry with them as they passed through the upheavals of China's efforts to modernize

over the forty years from 1949 to 1989? Where did they fit in
the scheme of 'New China'?

The challenge was to reconstruct these experiences in the
context of modern Chinese history, of modernization theory,
and of theories of cross-cultural relations. My hope is that,
enriched by the work of many scholars, this book offers the
reader a sense of the nature of the interaction between cultures, over time, and a clear view of how this author inter-
prets the significance of this encounter.

Research Method and Design

A longitudinal study of technology transfer at the West China
University of Medical Sciences (the new name given to the
Medical and Dental College in 1985) over an eighty-year
period examines the mechanisms and implications of cross-
cultural technology transfer by focusing on the medical
alumni trained at this institution before 1949. The primary
interest of this research is to explore the process of technology
transfer and diffusion to an indigenous group over time. The
purpose is to show how this elite relates to the broader network of traditional and revolutionary values, development
trends, and policy-making in contemporary China.

Western social scientists conducting research in China have
a particular set of limitations to contend with. The experience
of cross-cultural research in other settings confirms the notion
that the 'detached, impartial, statistically focused model is
dysfunctional.'[3] It is more productive in the Chinese setting
for the researcher to adapt to the host culture, allowing some
distance from his or her own culture to facilitate comprehen-
sion of the subjects' perceptions and perspectives.

Since history is the confounding variable in understanding
the relationship between cause and effect in a longitudinal
study, the most useful approach has been what may be called
a 'naturalistic study,' where the researcher tries to make
conceptual sense of data from multiple sources (interviews,
observations, and documents) by organizing them into categories.[4] Working from a set of research questions, the researcher

then derives hypotheses from the data. The foreigner in China has always laboured under the restrictions of Chinese ethnocentrism and xenophobia and must constantly search for disconfirming evidence to avoid mistaken conclusions from incomplete or distorted evidence. However, a combination of valid, corroborative data and logical analysis ensures more reliable answers to research questions. In this study, the research is based on interviews, archival sources, and observations, each of which will be discussed in turn.

There is a rich archival record of the West China Union University at the United Church of Canada Archives at the University of Toronto. A thorough investigation of this source, complemented by interviews with Canadian medical missionaries, formed the foundation from which to study the Chinese record of this story. This archival source provided the missionaries' own records and perceptions of their goals, strategies, achievements, and failures in West China. The archives of the Department of External Affairs in Ottawa added a new dimension – the perceptions made by Canadian outside observers of the role of the missionaries in the broader context of Sino-Canadian relations. The American observers, whose perceptions are recorded in the China Medical Board Archives in North Tarreytown, New York, provide the valuable perspective of a group engaged in the same work as the Canadian medical missionaries, but operating in a different location, with substantially more funding and slightly different goals.

After a year of correspondence with the West China University of Medical Sciences, it was arranged that I visit Chengdu in 1986 to explore the possibility of studying the school's history. The culmination of the archival research in Canada and the United States would be to gain access to the archives in Chengdu. These archives were confiscated by the Communist government in 1951, and again in 1966 by Revolutionary Red Guards during the Cultural Revolution. In 1984 the Sichuan provincial government returned the archives to the university, on loan for the purpose of compiling a history of the school in preparation for its seventy-fifth anniversary. On

my first visit to Chengdu in the autumn of 1986, my request
for access to the archives was met by several delays, but eventually cardboard boxes of files arrived at my room in the university guest-house. These included student records, correspondence, calendars, annual reports, student theses, and
campus publications. They arrived shortly before my departure and allowed only a hurried perusal. I was promised that
I would be welcome to return to Chengdu to examine the
archives. On my return to Chengdu in the spring of 1988 and
again in the spring of 1989, I was allowed to work in the
archives.

The president and senior faculty of the West China University were interested in this research project. They had
commissioned an in-house publication of a pamphlet on the
school's history[5]. Other Christian universities in China had
been the subject of Western research,[6] and my research was
viewed as an opportunity to make the West China University
of Medical Sciences known abroad, thus enhancing opportunities for international scientific exchange.

The archives are housed in the Old Library building (*Lao
Tushuguan*) on campus, across the lane from a factory which
operates twenty-four hours a day, so it is a rather noisy and
dusty place. The staff were willing to let me move files, a
table, and a chair to an upstairs corner at the far end of the
building, where it was quieter. The power supply was unreli-
able, so I decided to work near a window where natural light
could augment the feeble electric light. The archival documents themselves are not housed in a protective environment,
and many are faded or worm-eaten or have disintegrated. The
fragile documents must be handled with great care to prevent
further damage.

The archivist acknowledged that I was the first foreigner
admitted to the archives, and the rules for my visit were unclear. Chinese researchers themselves do not have carte
blanche access to the files. The most difficult handicap was
the lack of any index, and I was not allowed to peruse the
'stacks.' Therefore, I presented a list of file names based on
conjecture. I explained my research goals to the archivist, and

the request produced a proliferation of documents. Most of these were photocopied, and some of the more fragile were translated on site. The files which I used included correspondence in English, minutes of meetings of the Board of Directors, annual catalogues, student application forms, student records, official correspondence between the university and various governments of China and Sichuan (including a handwritten note from Yuan Shikai, briefly president of the Republic of China in 1916), Religious Life Committee correspondence, alumni correspondence, thesis regulations and topics, *West China Pharmaceutical Association Newsletter,* 'Enemy Political Files' (compiled by the Communist Party as evidence of the university's imperialist links and anti-revolutionary activities), *West China University News* bulletins (1920s through 1940s), detailed curricula, the university's constitution, and applications for employment[7]. Availability of files depends on the director's judgment, the attitudes of his superiors, and the 'thirty-year ruling,' although these rules are not entirely clear. Since other researchers had had their notes confiscated, I was not confident about the outcome of this effort. However, only one document was recalled because it had been published in 1960, and was, therefore, still within the thirty-year ruling for confidentiality. Because of the university administration's regard for this research project, the archives office was supportive of my efforts, and I probably enjoyed a better reception than I might have had with a topic unrelated to their interests.

The most important goal of the first exploratory trip in 1986 was to identify the surviving medical and dental alumni of West China Union University, and to get some sense of how many there were and what had become of them after the Revolution of 1949. Late one evening, a distinguished white-haired surgeon arrived at my guest-house room with a list of pre-1949 graduates who are faculty members on the Chengdu campus. I had requested the opportunity to interview this group and asked that the list be grouped by address in order to facilitate the interview schedule. What I received was a list grouped by generations: the 1920s, 1930s,

and 1940s cohorts of West China's medical and dental
alumni.

It is not unusual to conceptualize the peculiarities of each
'generation' of Communist China's leadership, both political
and intellectual, as the 'fifties, sixties, seventies, or eighties
generation.' The pre-1949 elite, however, is frequently referred
to as just that. In fact, as the work of a number of scholars
suggests, each generation was influenced by its own historical
consciousness.[8] Each group was shaped by the political events
of a shifting power base and the opportunities and necessities
created by an unstable economic and military environment.
The tendency to conceptualize the pre-1949 intellectual elite
as a homogeneous group reflects their treatment by the Communists. They were branded as the bearers of Western, bourgeois, liberal thought. Their education and socialization were
anathema to the goals of socialist transformation of Chinese
society as conceived by the Chinese Communist Party. But as
the bearers of crucial technical expertise, this group was indispensable as the 'first generation' in building the New China's
system of higher education. A study of their characteristics,
based on extensive interviews reveals a more complex group
and suggests some of the factors that influenced their career
development and subsequent influence on China's medical
development after 1949.

From 1986 to 1989 I had the opportunity to interview forty-
four alumni in Chengdu, Leshan, Beijing, Tianjin, Shanghai,
Hong Kong, New York, and Toronto.[9] The initial interviews
were semistructured, beginning with a set of questions to
establish basic biographical data and followed by an open-
ended interview on family background, student life, individual
political history and professional career (usually inextricably
linked), and ideas about medical policy and education. This
first set of interviews was used to formulate a standard questionnaire,[10] which was used for subsequent interviews and
mailed to eighty-eight alumni throughout China. Where possible, members of the first contact group were revisited to fill
in data that had not been obtained in the first interview. The
research design, which combined questionnaires and inter-

views, allowed a survey of a geographically dispersed sample of alumni, as well as more concentrated contact with alumni in selected locations.[11]

The standard questionnaire was mailed in China in the proverbial plain brown envelope with no return address on the outside to identify it as originating from a foreign source. A stamped return envelope was provided so that the one-*yuan* return postage would not be a deterrent to returning the completed questionnaire. The form included a request for confidentiality, which could be signed at the subject's discretion. Some of the respondents were careful to withhold any information that could lead to their identification. The data are, therefore, incomplete, and the responses provide varying degrees of detail. The questions themselves often probed sensitive areas of memory and political security. The biographical nature of the questions was reminiscent of the numerous 'self-confessions' imposed on the alumni during successive political campaigns in post-1949 China, especially during the Cultural Revolution of 1966–76. This may have inhibited the response to politically sensitive questions.

Both the framing of the questions and the varying quality of the responses limit the usefulness of statistical analysis. However, a system for coding the answers was devised so that systematic analysis could reveal patterns and trends, which are reported in chapter 4 on the alumni. The archival data on student life, individual application forms, and faculty correspondence filled in many of the gaps in the questionnaire responses. The tools of survey research, combined with an in-depth qualitative analysis, provide a rich profile of the alumni at each stage of their professional development, from student to graduate to 'senior adviser' at China's hospitals and medical and dental faculties.

The research benefited from a relationship that was established over a four-year period. Each visit or interaction with the alumni allowed access to more information and more candid explanations. These often served to correct mistaken assumptions arrived at from previous research. In spite of the fact that the political atmosphere in China was 'open' during

the period of this research, the politically 'seasoned' alumni
were cautious, and it may be that their caution was borne out
by the events of June 1989, when the final data were collected
for this book. A very real dilemma encountered in this study
has been the sensitivity of some of the research data in com-
promising the security of the respondents. It is difficult to
assess who is the most reliable judge of this issue, an internal
participant or an external observer. A personal dilemma for
me is the poignancy of individual histories and the tendency
of a Western-educated intellectual to identify with the alumni. It is a challenge, and perhaps not entirely appropriate, for
any researcher to maintain a completely objective point of
view in a study which charts the range of human hope and
despair during such a tumultuous period of history.

1

The Framework

Foreigners in China

From the time of Matteo Ricci's presence in the Ming court in the early 1600s, Chinese ambivalence towards Western learning has influenced the Chinese response to that learning. Ricci's introduction of Western knowledge posed a challenge to the existing academic authorities, and it was initially rejected. Centuries later, medical missionaries in Sichuan faced the challenge of convincing the Chinese that the Christian religion was superior and that Western science, with its technological and cultural attributes, was the answer to China's drive for modernization. As the sole providers of modern medical care and education to a population of ten million in the Chengdu Plain of central Sichuan, their goal was to contribute to the transformation of an ailing China into a modern nation, guided by the principles of Christianity and the scientific method.

Western influence became a salient factor in China's modernization from the time of the first Opium War in 1838. Commissioner Lin Zexu was appointed by the Qing government to suppress the British opium trade, which was draining China of its silver reserves and ravaging its population with opium addiction. He advocated the adoption of Western military techniques to combat Western aggression.[1] During the Tongzhi Restoration of the 1860s, the Zongli Yamen, which was created to deal with foreigners, established modern ar-

senals, a translation school, and an office for the translation
of Western technological and scientific texts.[2] Zeng Guofan
and Li Hongzhang, high-level officials in the Qing administration of the late 1800s, modernized their provincial armies
using Western military techniques.[3] During the period of
national self-strengthening following China's defeat by Japan
in 1895, Zhang Zhidong advocated 'Chinese learning as the
essence; Western learning for practical use.'[4] This attitude
towards Western technology and learning characterized the
official Chinese approach to modernization in the nineteenth
and early twentieth centuries. The Chinese sought technological change, hoping to master 'barbarian techniques' to control
the barbarians, but they rejected institutional change and
feared ideological change that might infiltrate and destabilize
China along with the new technology.

This rejection was based, in part, on the traditional attitude
that alien cultures were inferior to the Chinese, and, in part,
on the threat that the new learning posed to the literati,
whose authority was vested in the study of the Chinese classics. The introduction of science as an optional subject for the
imperial civil service examinations had a profound psychologi-
cal effect on the intelligentsia, challenging for the first time
the intellectual foundations of Chinese society.[5]

The fundamental rejection of Western influence is apparent
when one considers the history of Western reformers in
China. Jonathan Spence has dedicated an entire volume to the
profiles of individuals who hoped to transform China through
the introduction of modern engineering, modern medicine,
Marxist revolutionary strategy, and modern military organization. O.J. Todd, Borodin, Galin, Chennault, and Bethune
were each used by the Chinese for their technological expertise, but they were never integrated into Chinese society because they were foreigners. Spence concluded that in spite of
foreign efforts to transfer technology with an accompanying
'ideological package,' the Chinese inevitably forced the Westerners to accept Chinese terms.[6]

In addition to the Chinese attitude to Western learning,
which they regarded as instrumental at best and as a threat to

Chinese society at worst, another obstacle to the acceptance
of foreign ideas and technology was the inability of the political system to support modernization efforts. The problem of
the administrative incompetence of the Qing, and later the
Nationalist, government led to the 'neutralization of the Western reformer.'[7] The inability of the political system to facilitate the absorption of new technologies and organizational
principles plagued famine relief efforts in the 1920s, and the
failure of the China International Famine Relief Commission
to build an infrastructure of roads, wells, and irrigation canals
to prevent future disaster illustrates the inability of a single
agency, particularly a foreign one, to solve developmental
problems of the magnitude of China's.[8]

The experience of Western reformers in nineteenth- and
twentieth-century China was characterized by several frustrat-
ing obstacles: the mistrust of foreigners, the fear of the challenge to established authority, the rejection of institutional
change, and the political incompetence of successive Chinese
governments to carry out reforms. But in spite of the frustration and failure often faced by foreigners in China, their efforts were not fruitless. Much has been written about the role
of missionaries in the modernization of China. Their contribution as the bearers of modern science, education, and social
reform has been widely acknowledged. John King Fairbank
refers to the missionaries' pioneering role in fomenting the
Revolution of 1949 and considers their schools, hospitals, and
universities as their legacy to the People's Republic of China.[9]
The missionaries began to interact with the Chinese 'as China's old order began to crack,' and this vulnerability to foreign
influence allowed the Protestant missions 'to make their
contribution to the Chinese revolutionary process.'[10] C.H.
Peake asserts that 'the introduction of Western science and
the application of its methods' constituted the first phase of
the transformation of China into a modern nation.[11] Harold
Lasswell observes that the scientific contributions of missionaries determined their role as agents of modernization in Asia:
'Christian missions in the Far East were more effective dis-
seminators of non-religious than of specifically religious fea-

pean civilization. Hence much of the credit for
the peoples of the East and stimulating their
gies must be given to the missionaries in their
ransmitters of the secular elements of Western
clusion suggests that the future impact of missionary effort is likely to be the same.'[12] Although the missionary enterprise in China failed in its goal to Christianize that
nation, its secular contributions have not been overlooked.
This emphasis in the literature on the secular aspects of missionary endeavour focused the present study on the role of
medical missionaries.

Ralph Croizier's study of the interaction of modern medicine and rising Chinese nationalism describes the introduction of Western medical practice in China by medical missionaries.[13] Missionaries trained the first Chinese practitioners
of Western medicine, and developed Chinese scientific terminology to allow the translation of Western scientific and medical texts. They introduced the hospital as an institution for
the care of the sick and the concepts of civic sanitation and
public health as measures to prevent disease. Croizier's study
points out that the fatal flaw in the missionary effort to introduce medical modernization was the absence of government
participation. It was beyond the capability of private and
religious organizations to support the escalating cost of modern medical institutions. In addition, medical modernization
required institutional and social change which the Nationalist
regime was unable and unwilling to undertake. Peter Buck's
study *American Science and Modern China* describes the
missionaries' major effort as an attempt to establish the authority of modern medicine, its institutions and its practitioners, in a society which traditionally ascribed a relatively low
status to physicians. To do this, they created an exemplary
system of modern medicine within the mission compound,
with 'the physician as a man of influence,' and the 'hospitals
... as islands of cleanliness and order in an unregenerate
society.' This 'mission-centric' orientation, and the assumption that the organizational principles and practice of scientific medicine were universal, placed the missionaries in an

intractable dilemma. Buck explains this conflict between missionary goals and Chinese reality: 'As with the conceptual problem of relating universal laws of natural order to an environment where departures from them were the rule rather than the exception, here, too, the issue was one of squaring judgements about necessary uniformity with the undeniable facts of social diversity.'[14] Other studies on the impact of Western medicine in China assess the sociopolitical influence of medical missionaries and their role in the diffusion of ideas and technology in the modernization of health care in China.[15]

The literature on the role of missionaries in other developing nations suggests that, like their counterparts in China, they were the primary agents in the diffusion of Western ideas and technology and that their impact was predominantly secular rather than religious. In the Polynesian Islands, medical missionary success in curing disease identified the missionaries as the purveyors of a superior culture and gave them godlike status.[16] In Barotseland, they introduced the Western concepts of progress, industrialization and urbanization through their medical and educational institutions, and they have been credited with contributing to the creation of Northern Rhodesia.[17] The literature on 'the missionary factor' in African national, social, and political development focuses on the impact of missionary education, social services, and medicine.[18]

While historians have long realized the importance of missionaries in social and cultural transformation, the political-science literature on development pays little attention to them. The political development literature mentions the role of indigenous elites, and more recent literature focuses on foreign aid and diffusion of technology,[19] but the process whereby external agents of change influence modernization has been inadequately studied. This gap in the literature on political development suggests that political scientists should examine the missionary experience to assess its consequences for political development.[20] The introduction of Western ideas and technology is a factor contributing to social and political change, and medical missionaries, who vigorously attempted to import Western ideas and technology into China with the specific intention of transforming that 'backward nation,' are an important focus for the student of modernization.

Chinese Re-evaluation of the Christian Universities

After 1950 the Chinese Communists focused on the negative role of the Christian universities in China. Their prominent role in the development of a modern system of education came under attack as an instance of imperialist cultural aggression. In addition to vitriolic attacks on the institutions, faculty, and alumni, many of the schools were disbanded and reorganized into universities and technical institutes along the Soviet model. In 1980, however, Chinese researchers began to delve into the history of these universities, cataloguing long-neglected archives, re-establishing links with Western educational institutions and researchers, and reassessing the role of the Christian universities in China's modernization.[21]

The assessment of Western education in China, from 1949 to 1980, was characterized by ideological rhetoric about 'U.S. cultural aggression.' In 1949, Mao Zedong wrote 'Farewell Leighton Stuart!', an exposition of the Chinese Communist perception of American involvement in China. From Mao's point of view, there was a close link between American military support of the Nationalists under Chiang Kai-shek to suppress communism, and American support for liberal-democratic education in the Christian universities. Leighton Stuart, born in China at the end of the nineteenth century, was a missionary who later became president of Yenjing University in Beijing. In 1946 Stuart was appointed American Ambassador to China, thus, according to Mao, embodying the link between U.S. 'cultural aggression' and U.S. military aggression in China.[22] Communist political education in the early 1950s was aimed at those Western-educated intellectuals, 'Chinese liberals or democratic individualists,' who held 'muddled ideas and illusions about the United States.'[23] American science and technology were perceived as exploitative tools of imperialism to 'oppress the people at home and to perpetrate aggression and to slaughter people abroad.'[24] Under the circumstances of American military support of the defeated Guomindang, and their economic blockade of the new Communist regime, Mao's hostility to American institutions is understandable.

Following the Open Door policies of 1978, Chinese researchers began to approach the history of Christian universities in a more objective manner, and they began to sift through the events of decades of Christian college activity in pre-1949 China, to evaluate the role of Christian-sponsored education in China's modernization. The first phase of this re-examination of China's links with the West has been to assemble the archives of the thirteen former Protestant and three former Roman Catholic universities. In a joint effort with Princeton University, funded by the Luce Foundation, this process has been linked to a cooperative effort with foreign scholars and archives since 1986.[25]

It has been increasingly acknowledged that these missionary-run schools were an essential conduit for the introduction of modern methods of education and research into China. An evaluation of both the negative and the positive consequences of cultural interaction marks the search for greater objectivity in assessing the role of missionary colleges in China's modernization.[26]

The Role of Intellectuals in China's Modernization

Ultimately, the study of cross-cultural technology transfer must focus on the recipients, in this case the Western-educated medical elite. Their role must be understood in terms of the broader role of intellectuals in China, including that of teachers, scientists and physicians. Based on the traditional interaction between intellectuals and society in China, what impact could such an elite have on China's modernization? What characteristics of the Communist system influenced their fate as purveyors of modern medicine in a modernizing China?

The politics of modernization have defined the role of China's intellectuals since the late 1890s. The state's desire to control the transmission of ideas and values, and the application of knowledge, was fulfilled in the traditional Confucian system, where intellectuals were subservient to the political leadership and instrumental in legitimizing and implementing political authority.

With the radical changes in 1949, however, the Chinese Communist Party was caught in the dilemma of relying on the expertise of the intellectuals while rejecting their values. Determined to control those in the strategic role of transmitters of knowledge, the state imposed control on the pre-1949 generations of intellectuals, attempting to circumscribe their autonomy and authority. The extent and methods of control fluctuated over the decades between 1949 and 1989, with varying degrees of severity. These 'cycles of relaxation and repression'[27] culminated too often in a series of anti-intellectual campaigns: 1942, 1948–9, 1951, 1954, 1957, 1958, 1962, 1964, 1966–9, 1973–4, 1979, 1981, 1983, 1987, and 1989.[28] A 'two-line struggle,' between 'redness,' or ideological purity, and 'expertise,' tossed the scientific elite back and forth between conflicting political factions within the Communist Party. The overwhelming variable defining the lives of the intellectual elite has been the political environment in China, from the Qing dynasty's decline to the Open-Door policy of the Communists' modernization drive.[29]

The intellectuals have been defined by two elements: their role and their class. David Apter, in The Politics of Modernization, describes role as 'a functionally defined position in a social system. It embodies norms of conduct and expectations of action.' Class is defined as 'a multibond group that is the product of converging dimensions such as occupation, income and education.' In the process of modernization, Apter suggests that the modernizing scientific elites depend on free access to information, verification, experimentation, and empiricism. Their eligibility is based on technical expertise. Moreover, they tend to accept 'whatever political system they find in their societies,' motivated primarily by their need for information. In most cases, Apter states, '... the scientists in modernizing roles are supported by the universities, and universities in modernizing countries are often the focal points of liberty.'[30] In the case of Communist China, however, the intellectual autonomy demanded by the role of the scientific elites as modernizing intellectuals was in conflict with the Chinese Communists' desire to control the sources of information and the limits of professional autonomy. Although the Chinese Communists were dedicated to eradicating the bourgeois class, which is how they categorized the intellectuals in the early years of their rule, they could not afford to eradicate the role of professional bearers of scientific expertise critical to a modernizing society. The contradiction between a role that was at the pinnacle of the social order, and a class that was at the bottom, resulted in the conflicting treatment of intellectuals over the next half century. The alumni of Christian universities in China were in the untenable position of being Western-trained bourgeois intellectuals, anathema to the value system and class stratification of the new Communist state, but in the critical role of scientific experts and teachers, indispensable to the building of a modern state.

Under the Chinese Communist Party, intellectuals were 'singled ... out as specialized carriers of ideological and social initiative, but also as harsh enemies kept out of the proletarian fold and ruthlessly suppressed.'[31] Gordon White, in his study of the political role of professionals in China, captures the inherent dilemma of the relationship between the party/state and professional teachers. 'Exalted university professors,' he states, are on the one hand 'the jewel in the diadem of socialist construction.' On the other hand, they have 'implicit power which accrues to them from their distinct occupational role: as transmitters of the social values and expertise crucial to China's socialist modernization.'[32] If the party demands control of values and expertise, it is potentially in conflict with those who possess knowledge and are in a position to disseminate it. This of course characterizes the relationship between technical experts and the Communist Party. As Denis Simon points out in a discussion of China's scientific elite, they have posed a threat to the political elite since the late 1890s,[33] when politics and science struggled with each other to dominate the modernizing process. This struggle between political control of scientific education and research is illustrated many times in the intellectual history of the years between 1949 and 1989. Lawrence Schneider, in his study of Lysenkoism in China, points out that the acceptance of Soviet science as a symbol of the rejection of American-Western science and politics resulted in the stifling of scientific progress in genetics research for decades.[34] Like the geneticists in post-1950 China, the Western-trained medical elites were prevented from achieving their potential contribution to the development of medical research, education, and service in post-1949 China.

State control of education is not a recent phenomenon in China. Intellectuals have been considered instrumental in the pursuit of political goals for centuries. To seek examples from this century, however, we can refer to Zhang Zhidong, 'the chief architect of the new school system' in the early 1900s. In 1903 Zhang's Principles for the Control of Schools restricted students to academic pursuits, censored unorthodox texts, and tried to censor politically inflammatory language. Words such as yundong (movement) and daibiao (representative), so much a mainstay of contemporary Chinese political vocabulary, were excluded from acceptable usage. After 1905, when the civil service examinations were abolished, the state lost control over the upward mobility previously granted by state-controlled education. As Borthwick notes, the link between scholarship and officialdom was dissolved.[35]

During the republican era (1911–49), science and technology became instrumental in China's search for wealth and power. It was also the entrée to the international community. From 1927 to 1945 two generations of professional scientists emerged, trained in the Western system. They enjoyed relative autonomy in the universities, unencumbered by a weak political system, which initially was struggling to establish its control over all of China and subsequently was thwarted by the Japanese occupation.[36]

After 1950 the ideological constraints of the Soviet model combined with the traditional pattern of intellectuals subservient to the state, each pattern reinforcing the other. In 1956 the intellectuals were reclassified as more politically acceptable mental workers. Zhou En-lai, in an attempt to recapture the dwindling enthusiasm of intellectuals beleaguered by an excessive administrative burden, political interference with research priorities, and inadequate infrastructure to support teaching and research,[37] admitted that most intellectuals were 'progressive,' and political thought reform was more important than their class background. This allowed some improvement in the political status of professionals. By the end of the Cultural Revolution, in 1976, however, the rabid anti-intellectual wave that had swept China for ten years left the intellectuals, and teachers in particular, as 'virtual Gullivers, pinioned from many sides by a variety of political forces: PLA [People's Liberation Army] or worker propaganda teams, students, mass organizations, newly recruited or rehabilitated administrative and political cadres, and outsider mass management committees.'[38]

The Four Modernizations enunciated in 1976 and the concomitant Open-Door policy in 1978 reasserted the pivotal role of technological elites in the modernization process; however, they now had to overcome the obstacle of entrenched political power of the ideological elite. The resentment of those in power was further fuelled by the opportunities available to technical experts to travel abroad and earn extra income in a more open skills market.[39] The resistance to and fear of Western political ideas that contaminated Western technology led to the candid statement in the People's Daily that 'decadent and degenerate ideology and culture will enter our culture along with science and technology.'[40]

To instrumentalize the scientific elite, and indeed the entire intellectual class, the Communist system ensured that they had no autonomous social base to grant them political influence or power. From the 1950s to the 1980s, they functioned exclusively within the state structure, with no autonomy to organize or express their ideas. Beginning in the early 1980s, intellectuals were granted a degree of freedom to associate for professional purposes; they held conferences, formed alumni groups, and developed horizontal lines of communication, but no political expression was tolerated.[41] As in the Yenan days, the early days of Communist rule, and the first few years of the post-Mao modernization drive, intellectuals were encouraged to participate in economic development, but regarded with suspicion for their political unreliability.

With the demands of modernization in the 1980s, the scientific and technological elite were needed to bridge the gap between the West and China in terms of economic development. This burden fell on the pre-1949 generations of intellectuals. As Denis Simon observes, 'due to the existing age structure of the scientific community, many of China's best-trained scientists are advanced in age ... they are still badly needed to ensure that quality standards are maintained within the research system.'[42] After decades of abuse, however, Deng Xiaoping's 'mental labourers of the socialist working class' were 'weary partners in this renewed alliance.'[43]

According to William Kirby, the political controls imposed on the scientific and technological intellectuals in Communist China led to a truly 'poor and blank' record of development during the Maoist period. The 'new generation of internationally minded technocrats' are still hampered by political mistrust of their professional autonomy. In spite of the continuing conflict between political control and professional autonomy of China's scientific elite, the People's Republic of China is still left with the legacy of Goumindang China: 'personnel, experience, and precedents' in the presence and influence of the Western-educated scientists who staffed research institutes and universities after 1950. Years of political indoctrination and suppression marginalized their contributions to economic modernization, but as Kirby concludes in his assessment of the Nationalist legacy, 'institutional patterns have been known to survive tyrants as well as incompetents.'[44]

While Cheek and Hamrin's study of China's establishment intellectuals reveals an integration of traditional Confucian elite culture with Leninist intellectual culture, both of which stress subservience to the state, the cohort in this study – the medical and dental alumni of West China Union University – is strongly defined by the added dimension of Western, Christian, and scientific education. Their combined biographies, studied in the context of Chinese political and social development, provide a profile of an extended generation of medical elites – the 1920s, 1930s, and 1940s, – and their role in China's modernization. Not establishment intellectuals, they were technical specialists, instrumental to the party's goals of modernization. Trapped between the parameters of the two-line struggle between red and expert, and characterized by both traditional and liberal Western values, they existed 'between two cultures.' As Apter observes about the process of modernization in a mobilizing society such as Maoist China, 'party politicians and technical experts' would come into increasing conflict as they competed over decision-making authority. He states that the modernizing process challenges the society's 'ability to integrate the two competing and antagonistic groups, the political elite and the technical, managerial and intellectual modernizing group.'[45] Clearly, China has experienced deep conflict and limited success in integrating the modernizing intellectual elite into Communist society. The survival and persistence of the pre-1949 scientific elite is a phenomenon of the long-term implications of cross-cultural technology transfer. The story of the interaction between the medical missionaries, as transmitters of Western science and technology, and the alumni of the WCUU College of Medicine and Dentistry, as the receivers of this knowledge, sheds light on the process and consequences of the international transfer of technology.

2

The Setting: Sichuan Province
and the Mission Stations

Sichuan Province is far from China's coastal cities. In spite of its natural wealth and productivity, it seems frozen in time, a remnant of Old China, far from the influences from abroad which have shaped the international character of cities like Shanghai, Tianjin, and even Beijing. The Yangzi River, which winds its way for more than a thousand miles from the interior of Sichuan to Shanghai, was marked by deep, unnavigable gorges. Until recent times, river boats relied on the muscle power of hundreds of coolies to drag the vessels through narrow gorges in the river. Even the subsequent development of river transportation and accessibility by air from the other major cities in China have not completely altered the sense of isolation that one feels in China's far western province.

It is this sense of remoteness which makes it all the more astonishing to come upon the campus of the West China University of Medical Sciences, a sprawling institution in the southern part of Chengdu, the province's capital. The campus is grand in its conception, covering hundreds of acres, landscaped by flower-lined walkways, trees, and a lotus pond bordered by a covered walkway, designed to inspire meditative thought. The buildings are a curious blend of British university architecture and graceful Chinese traditional structures. The Administration Building, with its red pillars, wide stone steps, and gently sloping eaves, is the centrepiece of the university's architectural beauty, and it dominates the central

avenue that runs through the main part of the campus. Although the interiors of many of the old buildings are dilapi-
dated, one is struck by the magnitude of the ambition of the
missionaries who built this place almost a century ago.

It was inconvenient to travel to Chengdu in the 1980s.
Travel within Sichuan Province is slow and tedious, with
poor roads, incomplete railway networks, and limited air
routes linking the cities and towns within the province. It is
extraordinary to contemplate the imagination and undaunted
determination which must have inspired nineteenth-century
missionaries, part of a World Evangelization movement, as
they set out to establish the network of schools, hospitals,
and churches of the West China Mission.

The United Church of Canada and West China

By the end of the nineteenth century, most of the coastal areas
of China had been occupied by missionary groups who had
established their schools, churches, and hospitals in the acces-
sible treaty ports. Canada came late to this venture, and found
a vast area for potential influence in West China, beyond the
deep gorges of the Yangzi River. In 1888, the Reverend Virgil
C. Hart of the Methodist Church of Canada described Sichuan
as 'an empire in itself, with its teeming millions.' The missionaries' goal was to bring the benefits of their religion and
civilization to the masses of Sichuan. Far from the established
missions in China's coastal treaty ports, West China was
almost virgin territory, to be conquered by a pioneering mission. Hart was enthusiastic about the possibilities for a Canadian missionary enterprise: 'Only think of the opportunity
God has given me to establish another mission and for
Canada!'[1] Later missionary statements echoed Hart's enthusiasm about the opportunity to establish Canadian Christian
influence and the importance of Sichuan as a strategic centre
for the development of their mission. Described as 'China's
largest, most populous, wealthiest, most strategic province,'[2]
it was destined to exert a 'great influence upon neighbouring
provinces of China and upon the spread of Christianity in

Thibet [sic] and other parts of Central Asia.'[3] During a time
when China was undergoing profound political change, the
missionaries believed that the impact of Western civilization
in Sichuan would reach beyond its borders: 'As goes Szechwan, so goes China.'[4]

Missionaries at the West China Conference in 1898 at Chongqing had decided to divide the province into spheres of influence in order to avoid rivalry and duplication of efforts. The
then-titled Methodist Mission of the Canadian Methodist
Church[5] was assigned an area of 20,000 square miles in the
province's heartland. This densely populated area known as
the Chengdu Plain is the most arable land in an otherwise
mountainous province. Traversed by the Min River, the Yangzi River, and the Yangzi's major tributaries, it has an extensive riverine transportation system for its many and varied
natural products. Outside the concentration of people in the
two main cities of Chengdu and Chongqing, the former a political and cultural centre and the latter a commercial centre,
the population was diffused, with ninety per cent living in
rural areas.

While Sichuan had excellent river transportation, the numerous market towns were connected by poor and frequently
hazardous roads, and railways were all but non-existent. According to V.C. Hart's report in 1888, 'There is no very great
concentration of wealth, as the largest cities are not equal in
population and trade to many of the Eastern and Northern
cities; neither do we find as much poverty as in other sec-
tions of China. There is perhaps a more even distribution of
wealth ... many millions are engaged in commercial and
manufacturing pursuits, yet the larger portion of the population is engaged in petty agriculture so generally practised in
China.'[6] During the half century in which the West China
Mission occupied this region, the rural area flourished commercially, but it never achieved significant economic modernization.[7]

Between 1892 and 1913 the West China Mission established ten central stations and eighty-one outstations. The
Methodist board's policy of concentration was reflected in

the strategically located central stations, each with access to hundreds of surrounding marketing towns and each equipped with a mission hospital or dispensary. By 1910 the mission had 'accepted the responsibility for the evangelization of 10,000,000 in West China ... equal to twice the Protestant population of the Dominion of Canada ...' Its territory included '26 walled cities, over 1000 market towns, and tens of thousands of small country villages.'[8]

Each of the carefully selected central stations was a focus of political or economic activity: central market towns surrounded by a network of market towns and rural villages, and county towns housing the district magistrate. By 1922 each of these ten cities was served by a post office, and Chengdu was designated the 'District Head Office' for the postal service.[9]

Chengdu, Chongqing, and Ziliujing (Zigong) were the largest stations, with the most well developed medical service. The seven smaller stations included Jiading (Leshan), Rongxian, Renshou, Pengxian, Luzhou, Zhongzhou, and Fuzhou.[10] The following brief descriptions of these ten stations set the context in which the missionaries established their institutions. These station sketches indicate the strategic considerations of geographic location, economic importance, and population distribution that influenced missionary decisions in their 'occupation of China,' and the factors that affected the success or failure of the various mission stations in establishing missionary influence.

Chengdu

The walled capital city of Sichuan Province, Chengdu, is centrally located in a vast fertile plain. The Chengdu Plain is densely populated by thriving market towns and small cities. Chengdu's population by 1920 was half a million, with another half million inhabiting the surrounding area. The city served as the administrative, cultural, and educational centre of the province. As the training centre for government officials, it spread its influence throughout Sichuan. Chengdu is rich in historical and religious lore and relics. It is also the com-

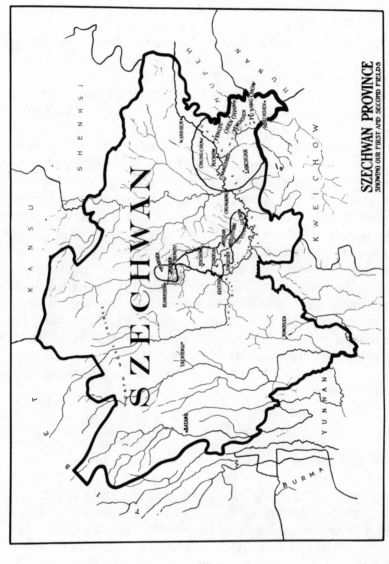

Map 1 Mission stations in Sichuan Province, from T.E. Egerton Shore, *A Statement of Mission Plant Required by the Canadian Methodist Church in West China and Japan, 1910*

mercial hub of the province, and the main trade and political link with Tibet.

The West China Mission was one of eight Protestant mission groups working in Chengdu. The mission established its first church in the Si Sheng Ci Temple district, near the city's East Gate. At the turn of the century, this area was relatively poor, but as the city developed commercially, so did Si Sheng Ci. The mission's strategy was to focus its efforts on the affluent and youthful members of the community. It chose to develop its second church in the centre of a neighbourhood inhabited by wealthy merchants and officials.

The medical work, originally intended to provide care for the foreign missionaries and their families, eventually expanded into a network of hospitals. The West China Union University, of which the West China Mission was a founding member, was also located in Chengdu, and therefore had the potential to exert influence throughout the province by educating Sichuan's elite. As mission resources diminished in the 1930s and 1940s, efforts were concentrated on the central institutions in the city of Chengdu. It is the university that has survived as the legacy of West China Mission work in Chengdu and that is discussed at length in chapter 3.

Chongqing

Chongqing was the commercial centre of Sichuan Province. It was a busy port at the junction of the Yangzi and Jialing rivers, and in 1916 its population was 700,000.[11] In spite of its commercial importance, the city itself was squalid and disorganized until 1937, when the Guomindang made it the wartime capital of unoccupied China and attempted to modernize the city. The early Canadian missionaries described it as the 'dirtiest and most unsanitary city of China.'[12]

The north bank of the city was the crowded Chinese sector, with thousands of steps up and down its steep slope to the river, prohibiting vehicular traffic. The south bank of the city was inhabited mainly by the foreign community: consuls, international commercial offices, gunboats of the imperial powers, and foreign missionaries, including the West China Mission and its business agency.[13]

The combination of hot, humid summers and open sewers running through the streets made Chongqing particularly unappealing to the foreign community. During the Sino-Japanese War, when the Canadian embassy was situated in Chongqing, Ambassador Victor Odlum found the city's atmosphere a great hardship. Among his many missives to Ottawa was a 1943 note that clearly stated his loathing of the city: 'I just want to throw up when I think of eating or drinking. Chinese slum habits are disgusting.'[14]

In addition to the physical conditions in the city, an early missionary noted the tension which existed between the Chinese inhabitants and the foreign community. Dr. Ed Cunningham, later a prominent professor at the West China Union University in Chengdu, wrote of Chongqing in 1925: 'Chungking is a treaty port and there are always gunboats there, this makes the Chinese mad. There are also a great many business people there, many of whom treat the Chinese badly and that makes them mad. It is a cosmopolitan city with people from all parts of China and abroad, many of whom are malcontents ... it has always been noted in this province for its bad atmosphere, as it were.'[15] In spite of these problems, the Canadian mission in Chongqing took over the old London Missionary Society Hospital in 1910 and eventually won the confidence of the Chinese inhabitants of the city.

Ziliujing

Outside of Chengdu and Chongqing, the Ziliujing (today known as Zigong) station was located in the most productive, densely populated city in Sichuan. The city, whose name means 'self-flowing wells,' was the centre of salt production in the province. Controlled by the National Salt Administration, it was a lucrative source of revenue for the central and provincial governments.

The Salt Administration dominated the political and economic life of the region. The central government's monopoly on salt dated from the Han dynasty (202 BC – 220 AD), and Ziliujing was the primary source of salt revenue. Yuan Shikai, the first president of the Republic after 1911, secured the 1913 Reorganization Loan from foreign sources using the salt monopoly as collateral. Yuan then had to agree to foreign administration of the *Gabelle*, and from 1913 to 1922, the tax was collected so efficiently that it exceeded the Maritime Customs revenue. This system was appropriated by provincial militarists after 1922, as they competed with the central government for control of Sichuan.[16]

The salt economy was characterized by a complex structure of producers who ran the wells, merchants who enjoyed semi-official status, and negotiators with the Salt Administration officials.[17] The missionaries recognized the importance of relations with this hierarchy, and their correspondence frequently refers to the various titles of the *Gabelle*: Salt Inspectorate, Salt Office, Salt Administration, and Salt Bureau.

The Protestant missionaries were not the first to seek to influence the gentry of Ziliujing. By 1870, a Roman Catholic mission had been established, and when Virgil Hart investigated the potential for a Methodist mission station in 1890, he was met with violent opposition from the local gentry and officials. They resented the foreign encroachment on their authority, and it was not until the suppression of the Boxers in 1900 that official sanction was granted to the Methodist mission.

Jiading

Jiading (Leshan), at the junction of the Min and Tong rivers, was the second station established by the mission, in 1894. It was both a religious and a commercial centre. Pilgrims streamed through the city, past the Giant Stone Buddha, on their way to the sacred Buddhist shrines of Mount Emei. Because of this strong Buddhist presence, the missionaries considered Jiading 'the hardest nut to crack in our present mission field.'[18] It was believed that the Giant Stone Buddha

overlooking the city intimidated many Chinese who might
otherwise have shown an interest in Christianity.[19]

In addition to its religious importance, Jiading was also the
centre for sericulture and silk weaving. As the upstream end
point of navigation on the Yangzi, it served as an important
trading centre for wood, musk, herbal medicines, and a native
white wax that was in demand in the European market.[20]

Although the gentry had steadfastly refused to sell land to
the mission, Dr A.J. Barter succeeded in securing the site of
an old temple on which to build the hospital, after he cured
the chief magistrate of malaria. Dr A. Stewart Allen, who was
later stationed at the hospital, relates the story that the
owner, having sold the property to foreigners, promptly put a
curse on it, condemning all future occupants to have only girl
children, a prophecy that was apparently true for the families
of all medical missionaries subsequently stationed there.

It is interesting to note that the hospital, built in 1924, is at
present part of a large medical complex that serves as the
county hospital. The original buildings, including the missionary doctor's residence, are used as medical wards and have
undergone only minor renovations since the withdrawal of
medical missionaries from Jiading in 1948.

Rongxian

Rongxian City was a walled town of 30,000 inhabitants in
1905, increasing to about 60,000 by 1940. It served as the
county seat and thus was the administrative centre for forty-
eight market towns. The county was rich in agricultural production and was endowed with a natural irrigation system of
rivers, a salt-producing district, and some relatively progressive gentry dedicated to developing a modern school system.

Initially the local gentry resisted the establishment of a
Protestant mission in their district. The Roman Catholic
mission had a history of interfering in local affairs, insisting
on extraterritorial rights for their converts. The magistrate
firmly opposed the intrusion of yet another missionary group.
Even the intervention of a prominent citizen, who had been

successfully treated for opium addiction at one of the mission hospitals, did not move the magistrate. Eventually, Dr W.E. Smith called on the magistrate, and presenting his passport, pointed out the treaty rights of British missionaries. It was 1905, just a few years after the suppression of the Boxer Rebellion, and the power of British gunboats was significant. Permission was granted to Dr Smith to purchase property on which to build the mission station.

Relations between missionary staff and Chinese staff were marked by a series of misunderstandings and conflicts during its history of almost half a century.[21] The hospital, however, did provide ongoing medical care for thousands of patients each year, with minimal staff. The hospital was closed in 1950, and its equipment was used to supply a new local hospital. One of West China Union University's earliest medical graduates, who practised in Rongxian, was executed by the new government in 1951.

Renshou

Renshou City, like Rongxian, was not an attractive site for missionary settlement. It was a secluded place, plagued by bandits and warlord armies, making road travel in the district unsafe. However, Renshou served as the central agricultural town for a population of more than one million, in seventy-five market towns, and thus offered the opportunity for enhanced missionary influence.

When Dr Smith surveyed the area in 1900, he was puzzled by the apparent enthusiasm of the gentry. He soon learned that they hoped to balance the overbearing influence of Roman Catholic missionaries in local affairs with a Protestant counterweight. Using this opportunity, the West China Mission established its station in Renshou in 1905.

The early missionaries described the town as 'a small, poor, mean-looking place, with much more than its share of moral blight even for a city in China.'[22] Although it was a busy market town, it was not on a waterway and thus was isolated from political currents which affected other parts of the province. Nonetheless, when the anti-Christian movement swept the country in 1926, the missionaries made their way to the Yangzi River to board British gunboats, which took them to the shelter of the foreign concessions in Shanghai.

When the hostilities abated in 1927, the mission elected not to station a foreign doctor in Renshou. In 1939, Dr Ralph Outerbridge was assigned to re-establish the clinical work, and the Canadian School, under Dr Lewis Walmsley, housed missionary children away from Chengdu, where threat of Japanese bombing was greater than in Renshou. Although the mission continued to support Chinese physicians in the medical work at the mission station, the support was minimal, and the station remained peripheral to the mission's medical work.

Pengxian

Located just a short distance northwest of Chengdu, Pengxian was an attractive residential town which served as a county seat for a population of one or two million. It was established as a mission station in 1897 to serve as 'a feeder to the big hospitals, schools and college already being planned.'[23]

Like Renshou, the station was evacuated during the anti-Christian movement, and few foreign doctors returned there after 1927. Because it was located so close to Chengdu, extensive medical facilities in Pengxian would have been impractical from the mission's point of view. The medical work never developed beyond a modest dispensary, in spite of the success of the early medical work.

Luzhou

Luzhou was in the centre of the West China Mission's territory, equidistant from Pengxian to its northwest and Zhongzhou to its northeast. It was economically and politically important, as the distribution centre for salt and sugar and as the central town of a large *tao*, or circuit of twenty-five counties. It served as the seat of government for the circuit intendant and the county magistrate and was a manufacturing centre for various small industries.[24]

After the 1911 revolution, which overthrew the Qing government, an independent revolutionary government emerged in Luzhou for a short time,[25] and the town was considered to be the 'chief city of Southern Szechuan.'[26] The population of the district numbered 400,000, and Luzhou itself, with a population of 200,000, was the educational centre for a fertile agricultural region.

The mission station was opened in 1908 in a rented house that was reputed to be haunted by demons. The hospital developed slowly, and when the medical work was centralized in 1945 in Chengdu, Chongqing, and Ziliujing, the limited mission support was withdrawn.

Zhongzhou

Zhongzhou (Chungchou) was a small, secluded residential town surrounded by mountains and located two hundred miles east of Chongqing. It was the first mission station through which the missionaries passed as they travelled the treacherous Yangzi gorges to Chongqing. Populated by 'landed gentry, scholars and common labourers,' Zhongzhou was the county seat and educational centre for its population of 10,000 and the seventy market towns in the district.[27]

The influence of Confucian tradition was strong, and it was said that the examination halls of the Imperial civil service were located 'on the pulse of the dragon,' and that the legendary 'Capital of Hades' was in the neighbouring county, frequented by numerous pilgrims.[28]

From the arrival of the first Canadian missionaries in 1910, the county and town of Zhongzhou had a reputation for political instability. Bandits and soldiers frequently terrorized the inhabitants, and moreover, anti-foreign hostility occasionally erupted in violence. In 1926, at the height of anti-Christian demonstrations, the wife of one of the missionaries was murdered on the street.[29] After foreign missionaries were evacuated in 1927, mission work was suspended for three years, and no foreign missionaries returned. The hospital continued to function under a Chinese graduate of West China Union University College of Medicine and was apparently taken over by the local community.

Remote from the other mission stations, Zhongzhou was a lonely outpost for foreign missionaries. A medical missionary who served there until the evacuation of 1927 referred to a Tang dynasty poem to express the sentiments of an isolated foreigner in the midst of a hostile Chinese community:

> ... relegated to deep seclusion
> In a bottomless gorge,
> Flanked by precipitous mountains,
> Five months on end the passage of boats is stopped
> By the piled billows that toss and leap like colts.
> The inhabitants of Pa resemble wild apes; ...
> Among such as these I cannot hope for friends
> And am pleased with anyone who is even remotely friendly.[30]

Fuzhou

Fuzhou City, located at the confluence of the Yangzi River and its navigable tributary, the Wu, was an important transportation junction. It had already been established as an outstation of the London Missionary Society in the late 1800s, and was taken over by the Canadian Methodists in 1913.

Fuzhou was a commercial and distribution centre for the salt-producing region south and west of it. The city was densely populated by close to 100,000 inhabitants and was the county seat to 134 market towns in Fuzhou county and forty-eight market towns in adjacent Zhangshou county.

Although the town had a history of anti-foreign sentiment, the medical mission developed from a thirty-bed hospital in 1915 to a 100-bed hospital and nurses' training centre by the mid-1930s. Although Western medicine was well received by the community, the medical work remained under the control of foreign missionaries, and the local elite never undertook responsibility for the hospital. When the missionaries left in

1946, the hospital deteriorated until the change of regime in 1950.

Summary

This description of the characteristics of each of the original ten mission stations provides the context in which to understand early medical missionary efforts to change West China.[31] Mission policy vacillated between the desire to decentralize missionary efforts, covering as broad a territory as their limited resources permitted, and concentrating their efforts in the urban centre of Chengdu. The attraction of pooling resources within the university structure led to the centralization of medical efforts in Chengdu, much to the dismay of the more rural-oriented fundamentalists among the mission staff. It was the university and its affiliated teaching hospitals, however, that survived the violent political upheavals of twentieth century China. This institution established its roots in Sichuan's urban centre, and provided the foundation for West China's medical education and health care in the twentieth century.

Sichuan Politics

With its great wealth in agriculture, salt, textiles, and opium, and a population of sixty million in the 1920s, Sichuan was frequently a battlefield for political and economic control. The missionaries also recognized the challenge of winning Sichuan. Virgil Hart, in his survey of the area in 1888, saw the province's great potential as a strategic centre in the country: 'Secluded as it has been by natural barriers from that free intercourse with other provinces which electricity and steam are about to remove, it has remained up to the present time a sort of wonderland ... The past year has seen it introduced to North, East, and South by means of the electric wire, thus giving it politically all the privileges enjoyed by other provinces. Steam will tame the wild rapids of its mighty river, and bring an unimagined commercial prosperity to its wealthy centres ... it will become a highway of nations.'[32]

Although twentieth-century Sichuan was more in touch with events in the rest of China than it had been in 1888, it was not until the Japanese occupation of East China forced the Nationalist government to retreat to that province in 1937 that it became the hub of Chinese national development. Hart's enthusiasm was echoed by the missionaries, who, a half century later, envisioned the profound influence they could exercise on China's future from their strategic location in Sichuan.

The political instability of China was reflected in Sichuan. The parenthetical remarks of an early missionary best describe the political climate of the province before 1949: 'Politically the province of Sichuan is divided into five circuits (that is, when the province is sufficiently at peace to be considered politically)'[33] The Revolution of 1911, which ended dynastic rule in China, left a power vacuum in Sichuan after the collapse of the Qing administration. The abolition of the civil service examinations in 1905 had already seriously undermined the bureaucratic structure of the Imperial government, and confusion compounded disintegration as the avenues to political authority became unclear. The new political career pattern which emerged was military, as opposed to the civil-bureaucratic system which had existed in Imperial China, and a new generation of provincially oriented militarists emerged to grasp control of whatever regions they could. Sichuan was controlled by five major warlords: Liu Wen-hui, Yang Sen, Deng Xi-hou, Liu Xiang, and Tian Songyao. Like the warlords of North China, these men were described as oppressive, ruthless, cruel, and incompetent.

Under the Qing government, the province was theoretically divided into five circuits or *tao*, each one under the authority of an intendant who embodied the court of appeal for the magistrate's court. After 1927 the warlords had carved the province into five locally autonomous regions known as *fang qu*, or garrison areas.[34] Each militarist or warlord had his own elaborate bureaucracy with numerous petty officials. The bureaucracy was essentially powerless to carry out any of its functions except for tax collection. In some areas taxes had been collected twenty years in advance. The system, thoroughly corrupt, extracted revenue from the populace, but failed to provide any services. Even after the Nationalist government's consolidation of political control in Sichuan in 1938, the situation remained virtually the same. A report by a Western observer in 1947 indicates that in one of Sichuan's *xian* (counties), 90 per cent of the revenue was used to pay administrative salaries, while 6.39 percent of the county's income was divided among departments of health, social welfare, relief, reconstruction, education, and development projects.[35] The condition of local government was one of elaborate structure characterized by inefficiency and powerlessness. Provision for public welfare in the first half of the twentieth century was essentially non-existent.

Because of the constantly changing power structure of the province in the 1920s and 1930s, it was never entirely clear who maintained central political authority. The basic unit of government below the provincial level was the *xian*, which theoretically served as the link between provincial government and local units called *xiang* or *zhen*. These latter represented marketing towns or communities, and their officials carried out the extractive functions of tax collection and military and labour conscription. The Guomindang government attempted to exert greater control over the province after 1935 by instituting direct inspectorates or *qu* between the *xian* and *xiang* levels of government, but it is not clear that they served any consistent function.[36] The lowest level of political control was contained in the *bao jia* system, which was preserved from Qing times. The Guomindang attempted to revive the system after 1935 as the most effective means of local control. The *bao jia* was a system of mutual responsibility based on the organization of rural households into administrative units. Originally designed to register able-bodied males (*ding*) for purposes of military and labour conscription, the *bao jia* later assumed police functions of local self-defense and crime control, and in some cases tax collection.[37] Under the Guomin-

dang, the *bao jia* was used to monitor and suppress Communist activity.

The missionaries who attempted to reform Sichuan society
faced the challenge of identifying who the power-holders
were. Under the chaotic conditions of civil war, which pre-
vailed during most of the first half of this century, the organization of government varied from place to place and time to
time. The missionaries were required to recognize who the
authorities were: who would allow them to rent or purchase
land, to carry out epidemic control, to register their schools,
to provide financial support, and to lend them status in the
community. The missionaries interacted with two groups of
local elites: those in power, and those with influence. This
included political officials and their armed forces, and affluent
gentry.

At the local level, the *bao jia* system allowed the police to
identify everyone in the community, and the heads of each
family. This facilitated their effectiveness in carrying out
public-health measures, such as the supervision of vaccination
campaigns or the speedy burial of cholera victims.[38] Although
some of these measures were often initiated by the missionaries, they had no control over the means of enforcement.
General Yang Sen, one of the provincial warlords, was known
for his 'flamboyant,' if superficial, efforts to modernize his
region. In addition to widening streets and attempting to abol-
ish footbinding, Yang outlawed 'the raising of pigs in the
streets of Luchou,' and ordered the public beating of the city's
police chief for failing to enforce this prohibition.[39] In another
instance, military patrols in Chengdu were seen beating residents who left garbage in front of their houses.[40] The picture
that emerges from these descriptions of the local exercise of
power is that it was arbitrary and inconsistent.

In addition to government officials representing either militarist regimes or the central government, each town or village
had an acknowledged group of community leaders. The non-
official gentry class represented the wealthy landowners, merchants, or educated men of the district. One scholar attributes
their influence to the fact that they possessed 'social and per-

sonal prestige rather than ... any particular mandate,' and unlike government officials, were not the recipients of the official graft universally squeezed from government revenue.[41] In the 1940s this group was described as local 'gentlemen ... the current version of the Chinese gentry,' organized only in the sense that they shared interests, common socio-economic status, and bonds of friendship.[42] It was these men – members of the local Chamber of Commerce, wealthy merchants, school principals, Buddhist priests – whom the missionaries cultivated as valuable contacts to further the cause of their schools and hospitals in the community.

In addition to ensuring the survival and growth of missionary institutions in the 1920s and 1930s, missionaries sought to influence broader change by introducing to the local gentry the concepts of a modern health-care system and the universal right to medical care. They encouraged the public-spiritedness that had characterized the early development of hospitals in the West and appealed at the same time to the elites who had their own local agendas. In the mission stations outside the Chengdu campus of West China Union University, it was difficult to find elites who were both politically influential and who shared the same ideals as the missionaries. Missionaries who expected hospital board members to commit to the social, religious and political beliefs of a Western, Christian institution were frustrated by the clash of world views.

The missionaries were not always successful in soliciting support from this elite. When they first arrived in Sichuan in the late 1890s, Omar Kilborn described how they were despised by the local gentry: 'we were beneath contempt ... it was commonly supposed that we must have committed some crime in our own country, and that we were trying to escape the consequences by fleeing to this far interior province of their country.'[43]

The foreigners were expelled from Sichuan by anti-foreign, anti-Christian riots in 1895, by the Boxers in 1900, during the upheavals of the 1911 revolution, and by nationalist student-led hostilities in 1926. On each return, however, they gained some ground in their relations with the gentry. In 1896 local magistrates offered protection to the returned missionaries on orders from the Imperial court; in 1900 the threat of foreign gunboats on the Yangzi River subdued hostilities to missionaries and increased the scope of their activities under the protection of extraterritorial rights. After 1911, the newly formed republic was eager for foreign knowledge and technology. By the time the missionaries returned from their fourth expulsion, in 1928, the Nationalist government, which had consolidated control of the country from Nanjing, demanded devolution of foreign-controlled institutions to the Chinese. This spurred the missionaries to expand their contacts even further, in an effort to include Chinese elites on the boards of their institutions.

From the beginning of the Nationalist regime, then, the missionary institution became increasingly integrated into a modernizing society. The Guomindang, in its search for modern technology and administration, relied on the missionary teachers for the education of a modern intellectual and political elite. With this increasing interest came an increasing demand at least to share in control of foreign institutions. As nationalist sentiment increased, the demand for devolution of authority followed. In spite of some political tensions, the Nationalist period was the high point of Sino-Western relations, and the Christian universities, including West China Union University and its hospitals, were exuberantly bicultural.

The West China Union University College of Medicine and Dentistry

In 1914, in an era when China was searching for an educational model as a basis for its modernization efforts, the president of the new republic, Yuan Shikai, wrote an inscription to the newly founded West China Union University (WCUU). Its president, Dr Joseph Beech, received the following endorsement from Yuan: 'Nowadays, global communication has linked academic thought all over the world. Dr Beech's goal is to allow others to achieve this unity of culture and ideas. He stands at the forefront [literally, 'headwaters'] of this trend in establishing education in Sichuan.'[1] Beech and his colleagues in the West China Mission had an ambitious goal indeed: to contribute to Sichuan's modernization by linking it to the West through a Christian university. An early report of the General Board of Missions of the Methodist Church echoes Yuan's statement: 'Science may be said to have permeated the world when it has become an integral part of higher learning in as remote a spot as Chengtu, Szechuen.'[2]

The process of internationalization of education in China began in earnest at the end of the nineteenth century. Although China's traditional scientific elite controlled missionary influence in introducing Western science before 1840, many other avenues were opened after the Opium War,[3] including Chinese and foreign government scholarships to send Chinese students to Japan and the West to study engineering, medicine, and other sciences. Subsequently, foreign-trained Chinese scholars returned to China to teach in modern gov-

ernment and missionary schools. Perhaps the most established, and extensive, channels for foreign education in pre-
Communist China were the missionary schools, particularly
the Christian colleges, which trained several thousand Chinese students in the curricula offered by universities in the
United States, Japan, Great Britain, France, Germany, and
Canada.

The missionary colleges in China had as their goal not only
the evangelization of the Chinese, but the concomitant modernization that Christian missionaries associated with their
religion. Marion Levy described the missionaries' role as one
of modernizers in China.[4] The task that the missionaries set
for themselves was no mean feat: to modernize China single-
handedly by changing the country's moral fibre and social
norms and by introducing the best that Western science and
technology had to offer. The missionaries of the West China
Mission believed that China's salvation would lie in its acceptance of Christian morality and spirituality. Their emphasis, however, especially in the West China Union University, was on the secular aspects of Western civilization. The
introduction of modern science, especially modern medicine,
would provide the basis for China's transformation into a
prosperous and democratic nation. Their strategy of modernizing China 'from the top down' would be accomplished by
mobilizing the political elite to expand public responsibility
for health care. To allow government to expand its capacity
in this sphere, the missionaries would contribute medical
technology, institutions, and, above all, professional personnel
to carry on the development of modern medicine in China. In
the sphere of medicine, this group would be the 'modernizing
elite.' Armed with the goal of using science education to
develop China's future leaders, missionaries in the early 1920s
believed that 'the way opened up by this Christian university
will undoubtedly be followed by government institutions.'[5]

The political instability of Sichuan, however, militated
against the adoption of science for economic development by
local governments or even the national government at the
time. The Dean of the Medical College in 1935 characterized

Sichuan's successive governments as 'short-lived, and neither humanitarian nor humane.'[6] He forecast that under stable government leadership, the need for mission responsibility for medical care and education could eventually be phased out. Under such conditions, the goals of the university were to focus on training leaders for China's future development.

The stated goals of the WCUU College of Medicine and Dentistry were to train Chinese Christian physicians who would take over the institutions that the missionaries had built. These future leaders in medical modernization would teach in Chinese medical schools, staff Chinese hospitals, and serve as advisers to government ministries of health. In the interim, medical missionaries in West China concentrated on training this medical elite, building the physical and administrative infrastructure to provide medical care, and encouraging Sichuan's social and political elites to support the institution of a modern health care system.[7] Before 1949 medical missionaries at the WCUU College of Medicine and Dentistry measured their achievement by the growth of their institution, as estimated by the number of graduates, number of patients accommodated, and financial and political support from the Chinese community. Their long-term success would be achieved by transmitting to their students their own Christian, liberal-democratic values, and their knowledge of, and approach to, medical science, education, and care.

Description of the West China Union University

Although located in the heart of populous Sichuan Province, WCUU was a relatively isolated university, with limited resources and less outside influence from visiting scholars and new recruits than the universities in China's coastal cities. Situated in the provincial capital, Chengdu, it tended to be more conservative than schools in Shanghai or what was then called Peking; nonetheless, it exerted a significant modernizing influence in Sichuan and provided the only opportunity for many Sichuanese to receive a university education.

The university itself was founded in 1910 by five participating denominations, including the missions board of the
Methodist Church, later the United Church of Canada.[8] The
School of Medicine was established in 1914 with a faculty of
five medical missionaries, and an enrolment of seven Chinese
students. It doubled within a short period and continued to
grow and diversify. A department of dentistry was formed by
Dr A.W. Lindsay in 1917, becoming a college in 1919, and the
faculties of medicine and dentistry united in 1929 to form the
College of Medicine and Dentistry, under two separate deans,
but with one director as spokesman.[9] Dr Lindsay had originally been selected in 1907 for the purpose of taking care of the
dental needs of missionaries and other Westerners in Sichuan.
Inspired by the vision of training modern dentists for China,
Lindsay persuaded the board to recruit two more dental missionaries, Drs Thompson and Mullett, to form a faculty at the
university. It was agreed in 1929 that the medical faculty
would be a priority, and the ratio of medical students to dental students would be two to one. The impetus to elevate the
status of the dental program was the evacuation of missionaries in 1927. There was no Chinese professor of dentistry to
take over responsibility for the students, who consequently
transferred into medicine or science. To prevent further
setbacks to the development of a Chinese dental profession,
it was decided to concentrate on the training of future
teachers.[10]

As teaching became more specialized, a biochemist was
recruited to teach medical and dental students in their
preclinical years, and in 1930 Dr H.B. Collier established the
department of biochemistry within the College of Medicine.
This department was raised to the status of 'Institute' in 1948
as a bid for recognition and funding from the Nationalist
government in Nanjing.[11]

The Department of Pharmacy similarly grew from one pharmacist, Dr E.N. Meuser, who was originally assigned to man-
age the Chongqing Methodist Episcopal Hospital's dispensary
in 1910. In 1911 Meuser transferred to the Canadian Methodist Hospital pharmacy in Chengdu, where he urged the uni-

versity to establish a department in that field.[12] In 1917, the Canadian Mission School of Pharmacy was established with funds raised by Meuser from private drug companies in Shanghai, England, and the United States, and a matching grant from the university.[13] The secretary of the foreign missions board, Dr J. Endicott, opposed the expansion of the pharmacy program as part of the medical college,[14] but Meuser gained recognition for his department under the College of Science in 1932.[15] However, in 1941, the Department of Pharmacy was made a college in recognition of its important contribution to pharmaceutical research and manufacturing.

The College of Medicine and Dentistry was closely affiliated with the three West China Mission hospitals in Chengdu. Medical faculty staffed the hospitals, and the hospitals provided clinical instruction for the students.[16]

The WCUU was originally financed by the board of founders, whose office was in New York.[17] Administration was carried out by a board of directors in Chengdu,[18] and faculty appointments were decided by the individual mission boards.

The ethos of the university was one of integrating scientific and moral education. The university's code of conduct was embodied in an eight-character inscription naming virtues similar to the eight Confucian virtues of classical Chinese education: benevolence, knowledge, loyalty, courage, honesty, prudence, diligence, and harmony (see figure 1).

Perhaps because of the influence of the syncretism of Liang Shu-Ming[19] on China's intellectuals, the university's school song reflected the centrality of the cross-cultural interaction that was taking place on its campus:

> Europe and Asia intertwine;
> Two cultures embrace.
> Stately stands the Green Water Palace.
> From the Min mountains in the West
> Flows the scaled dragon.
> By its side the phoenix and unicorn.
> Hold fast our traditions
> To transform the world.

Extend our cultural roots;
Sustain the ideals forever.
The sages in the East
And those of the West
Together can reveal the Way.

West China Union University school song, circa 1920[20]

This song stressed the ethos of integrating ideas and values from East and West, to create a 'New Learning,' stronger than either culture's ideas and values alone. The challenge to the students was to strengthen their nation through both education and strong moral values. The balance between these two aspects of medical education was an ongoing issue in the development of the university's goals and policies over its forty-year history.

Education Models for the College of Medicine and Dentistry

In 1907, Omar Kilborn, the first medical missionary at the Canadian Methodist Hospital in Chengdu, reported the need

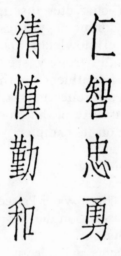

Figure 1 *Huaxi Xiehe Daxue Xiao Xun*. West China Union University school code of conduct, naming benevolence, knowledge, loyalty, courage, honesty, prudence, diligence, and harmony[21]

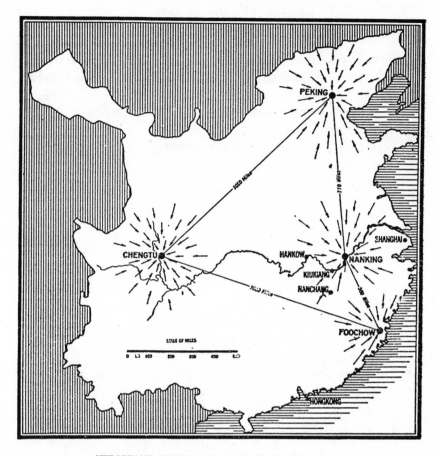

CHRISTIAN EDUCATION THE HOPE OF CHINA.
Strategic Christian Educational Centres. Union Universities are located at
Chengtu, Peking, Foochow, Nanking.

Map 2 The impact on West China of West China Union University, according to *Our West China Mission*, a summary by the missionaries in the field published in 1920.

for a cooperative medical school. Kilborn, who administered the hospital and served as physician, pharmacist, head nurse, evangelist, and teacher, wrote: 'I did just enough to realize the hopelessness of the "one-man medical school" as an adjunct to a large, busy hospital.'[22] This realization that a handful of missionary doctors could not hope to solve China's health problems, and the prevalent conviction that China must be evangelized 'from the top down' through its educated class, were the motives behind the establishment of a medical college in 1914 as part of the West China Union University.[23]

The rationale for providing professional medical education was the university's contribution to China's future development by serving as a 'strategic basis' for the solution of China's health problems.[24]

The justification for providing a university environment for medical education was given in the 1936 report of the special committee on policy: 'The wider background and greater detachment from the deadening effect of the immediate environment permit the medical missionary to supply a steady stream of vital Christian enthusiasm and scientific spirit ... Furthermore, the very great opportunity embodied in our Medical educational institutions for establishing the healing professions of whole nations upon Christian foundations is so challenging that the need for missionary medical educationalists is greater than ever before.'[25]

The College of Medicine and Dentistry was the largest faculty at the university and commanded the majority of the personnel and funding of the Canadian medical missionary enterprise.[26] Dr Leslie Kilborn, Omar Kilborn's son and his successor as dean of the college, pointed out that most of the staff were Canadians, and two wings of the medical-dental building were built with Canadian funds: 'Our Mission has always regarded this College as its very special sphere in this University.'[27] A report in 1939 explained the "unbalance"[sic] where medicine and dentistry have grown out of proportion to the other departments and faculties' as a result of 'the self-evident need of medicine, as well as the background of existing local medical practices.'[28] As early as 1926 the university's medical budget was ten times greater than that for the department of religion. This emphasis on medicine was not shared quite yet by the mission in general, whose 1928 budget for evangelical work still exceeded that for medical work.[29] There was some resentment on the part of the doctors who staffed the outlying mission station hospitals towards the inequality of funding and towards the university's attempt to monopolize the medical budget, to the perceived detriment of the station hospitals.[30]

In 1934 Dr J. Endicott, then the secretary of the foreign missions board, criticized the lack of cooperation from the participating mission boards in supplying funds and personnel to the university, as the cause for restraints on carrying out their programs. He noted that the burden always fell on the United Church of Canada (UCC), especially in the medical field, and that it was draining funds from the mission as a whole.[31] The support for medical education at the university was the most extensive commitment made by the UCC in this field. In their African missions, medical missionaries trained 'low-grade assistants'; in India, 'relatively little [had] been done towards medical education under mission auspices'; in North China, paramedical assistants were trained; and in Korea and North and South China, the UCC cooperated in supporting university medical schools. In West China, UCC not only cooperated in the support of the university and its medical college, but provided three of the four hospitals used for clinical teaching, the majority of the dental faculty, and a specialist in pharmacy and hospital technology.[32]

The model for medical and dental education adopted by the missionaries reflected their own goals and their own educational and professional backgrounds. The first call to the medical missionary to teach in a Christian medical college, put forth by Omar Kilborn, stressed the missionary's 'duty … to multiply himself by making medical missionaries among the Chinese.'[33] The medical college was organized to train leaders so that 'the multitudes of suffering men and women living in Sichuan and adjoining areas should receive the benefits of modern medicine.'[34] The missionary doctor was of value only to the extent that he could change the conditions of China's suffering on a large scale, and to do this 'he must be able to reproduce himself among China's young men.'[35] Thus the medical missionary, with his scientific medical training, professional code of ethics, and Christian spirit of service and self-sacrifice, was portrayed as the model for the development of a modern Chinese medical profession. Impli-

cit in this goal was the desire to produce medical educators
and administrators who would eventually take over the mission hospitals and medical college. Dr A.W. Lindsay, Dean of
the College of Dentistry, was more specific about the aims of
his faculty: 'To produce, in particular, dental staff for health
institutions, such as hospitals, health centres, public health
clinics, school clinics and the like; teachers and leaders for
public health service; dental administrators and teachers for
the dental colleges which are about to be organized throughout China.'[36] The dental faculty was more single-minded in
training teachers than the medical faculty, in part because it
did not have the dual objective of staffing a large network of
station hospitals and clinics as well as training medical educators.

In the pharmacy department, E.N. Meuser's objective was
to train Chinese students in the 'science of modern pharmacy'
and, at the same time, to 'develop systematic research in
Chinese crude drugs.'[37] In addition to the applied research and
professionalization of the Chinese pharmacist, Meuser envisioned his department as a model for pharmacy education in
China. William Band of the British Council visited the department in 1944 and reported: 'On the classroom walls is a large
map of the United States and Canada, showing the location of
pharmaceutical educational centres in North America. Every
student is encouraged to dream of a similar map for China.'
As for the manufacturing aspect of the pharmacy department,
Band described it as an attempt 'to combine Christian ethics
with modern business.'[38] Of the three professional schools,
Meuser's was the only one that candidly acknowledged the
remunerative aspects of the profession, and he attempted to
instill his values through practical application.

Before discussing the implications of these models of education for the college's curriculum, it is necessary to reiterate
the religious motivation behind these secular intents. Dr
Bruce Collier's goal in the teaching of biochemistry was 'to
relate Science to life as a whole, thus demonstrating its spiritual value.'[39] The rigours of teaching in Chinese as well as
administering a department and updating its technology made

it difficult for these teachers to spend time conveying their spiritual values. In addition, the conflict between science and the superstitious aspects of Christian religious belief was not lost on the students. A handwritten note inside a 1916 publication of the mission read: 'One of the greatest difficulties that seems perennial in my scientific work with the students seems to be the virgin birth of J.C. [*sic*].'[40] Most medical missionaries were so preoccupied with their teaching and clinical work that they had neither time nor inclination to evangelize, and, as illustrated above, the Christian message was not always consistent with the teaching of science. Many missionaries relied on personal contacts outside their teaching and clinical duties to transmit their Christian ethics, if not their religious beliefs.[41]

The organization of the university and the curriculum of the professional schools reflected the professionalization of medical and dental education in the West, and the predominantly University of Toronto background of the medical missionary group.[42] The 'Oxford Plan' used at the University of Toronto was adopted by the West China Union University, whereby denominational, autonomous colleges were responsible for 'all matters pertaining to the life of the students, except instruction.'[43] This organization reinforced the separation of evangelical and secular education at the University.

The curriculum for the medical college reflected the North American emphasis on basic sciences and hospital-oriented clinical training.[44] The United Board for Christian Colleges in China, a coordinating body of the thirteen Protestant universities, reported that the curriculum of the College of Medicine 'followed the general pattern of Grade A schools in the United States and Canada as laid down by the Association of American Medical Colleges.'[45] The medical course was seven years, with the first two being devoted to basic sciences and English.[46] Like the University of Toronto program, the last year of study included a 'clinical clerkship' in the hospital, followed by a one-year rotating internship. Following the University of Toronto's example, specialization was not allowed prior to attaining a general knowledge of medical practice during the internship year.[47] In 1932 Dr Leslie Kilborn required senior students to write a thesis.[48] By 1937 the college also offered a postgraduate diploma in ophthalmology and otolaryngology and a certificate in hospital technology,[49] developments indicative of the increasing scope and differentiation of the institution.

The dental curriculum was unique in that it shared the first two years of basic science training with the faculty of medicine, and it was also a seven-year course with a clinical internship in the university dental hospital. Like the medical curriculum, it adhered to the standards of 'Grade A' Dental schools in Canada. An observer from the Rockefeller Foundation's Peking Union Medical College remarked that the quality of teaching and curriculum exceeded that of medicine.[50] The WCUU integration of medicine and dentistry in the preclinical years was an innovation, designed to train scientific dentists rather than technicians. This followed the trend in Canada towards the professionalization of dentistry, but it was a departure from standard dental education in North America,[51] and more appropriate to the training of potential university professors of dentistry.

The pharmacy curriculum was four years in length and stressed basic sciences.[52] In addition, it promoted applied research into Chinese materia medica and taught technical skills.

Since students were encouraged to pursue postgraduate study abroad and to return to China as leaders in their profession, English-language proficiency was stressed during their training. To facilitate premedical studies, Chinese was the language of instruction in the first two years, after which English was gradually introduced.

Clinical teaching was carried out in the West China Mission hospitals in Chengdu. Together they had four hundred beds, and they treated two hundred to four hundred outpatients a day, providing the students with adequate opportunity to develop clinical skills. Instruction usually took place in small clinical groups of six to eight students, led by a staff physician who carried on bedside teaching. Students also participated in pathology rounds and clinical conferences, where the clinical decision-making process was elucidated through debate among staff and students. The small student-to-staff ratio encouraged extensive teaching, and in addition to patient-care responsibilities many students assisted in faculty research projects. Although the university was not as well endowed as its counterparts in East China, it endeavoured to train clinician-scientists to whom the teaching and administration of medical education could devolve.

In spite of the urgent need for physicians, dentists, and pharmacists in China, the University opted for an elitist model of medical education. The medical missionaries believed that their greatest contribution to China's development would be the training of men and women who could staff future medical colleges and thus maximize their influence. They rejected the alternative model, to train paramedics or lower grade doctors to provide for immediate need. There were no cogent arguments given for this decision to educate a small elite; the alternative model had in fact been the original means of training mission hospital assistants and was rejected as inadequate. Omar Kilborn's remarks in 1910 are indicative of the spirit of great institutions that inspired the medical and dental college: 'There is a general realization that the day of small things is over, and that larger and more thorough-going and more advanced work must be undertaken.'[53]

Institutional Development

In retrospect, the phases of institutional development of the College of Medicine and Dentistry can be divided into three periods. The first, from 1908 to 1927, was characterized by the primacy of evangelical goals enhanced by the provision of medical service to potential converts. The second, from 1927 until the outbreak of the Sino-Japanese War in 1937, was marked by the increasing secularization of institutional goals, as medical missionaries became more professional and less evangelistic. At the same time, China was united under the Guomindang government, which embarked on a decade of

modernization efforts and nation-building to which the missionaries had to respond. The influx of refugee universities
from East China after 1938 marked the beginning of the
period of institutionalization, from 1938 to the Communist
takeover of the university early in 1951, and resulted in the
transformation of the medical and dental college. As host to
Cheeloo Medical School, Peking Union Medical College
(PUMC), and National Central University Medical College,
WCUU enjoyed (and occasionally resisted) the expansion of its
faculty and its research and teaching capability. Challenges
to the traditional curriculum and teaching methods contributed to the increasing sophistication of the WCUU medical
program. The ultimate result of this infusion of ideas and
people from other regions of China was that the medical and
dental college exerted a wider influence through the postwar
distribution of its alumni than may have been expected from
such an isolated institution.

The goals of the medical college, which was originally separate from the dental college, evolved as the school grew
from an adjunct to philanthropic mission work into a professional institution. Among the faculty, however, there was
always an underlying debate about the appropriate goals for
medical education in Sichuan. PUMC represented the elite
approach to medical education, whereby clinician-researchers
were trained to the highest standards with the goal of developing China's future system of medical education. This was
held up by some as the model to which other medical
schools should aspire. In an editorial in the *Chinese Medical
Journal* in 1935, WCUU's dean of medicine, W.R. Morse,
expressed concerns that this model was inappropriate for
Sichuan, arguing that the missionary model was limited by
budget and staff constraints. Moreover, constant war, disease,
and hunger created a situation where 'fear is the commonest
disease amongst the laiety.'[54] By 1935 the university had
produced eighty graduates in medicine to serve a population
of sixty million. The military medical school in Chengdu,
which was staffed by French military surgeons, had closed,
and a competing private medical school in Chengdu, staffed

by several WCUU graduates, was described as an inferior institution.

Under such conditions as chronic underfunding, harsh living conditions, and the absence of other sources of medical education, Morse was convinced that the college's obligation was to train general practitioners, not scientists or specialists. 'The basic motif of our education,' he wrote, 'is the social service of medicine.' His ambition was not that the mission school be powerful or national in scope, but that it emphasize the training of doctors of high moral character. His formula for the ideal graduate was a general practitioner who was 'a scientifically trained, emotionally controlled artist.' He viewed the college as a 'technical vocational school to teach the art of applied science to medicine and dentistry.'[55] The college was at that time an undergraduate institution, and the isolation of graduates, once they went into private practice or missionary hospitals outside the major cities of Chengdu and Chongqing, made it essential that they be trained in problem-solving, and the skills for self-education, to carry on a general practice with limited technological support.

As thousands of refugee students flocked to Sichuan after the Japanese invasion of China in 1937, more cosmopolitan students and faculty joined the ranks of the medical college.[56] The three medical schools, Cheeloo, PUMC, and Zhong Da (the National Central University) were housed on the West China campus. They united their efforts in 1938 to form a medical training program inspired by the PUMC model. Based on the Johns Hopkins model of the medical scientist, it was the catalyst that encouraged the development of graduate training at the college. A residency program in the ear, eye, nose, and throat (EENT) specialty developed under Drs Peterson and Cunningham and was devolved to Dr Eugene Chen in the early 1940s.[57] The professional development of the curriculum and postgraduate training were no doubt fuelled by some competition with the government's National Central University, whose students and faculty looked down on the parochial nature of WCUU and the subordination of Chinese students to foreign faculty. The dean of medicine in 1943, Dr Leslie Kil-

born, was a generation younger than Dr Morse. His doctoral
training in physiology predisposed him to favour the development of medical research in conjunction with clinical training.
Kilborn lobbied the mission board, the Chinese government,
and American and Canadian funding agencies to develop postgraduate education in the medical college, and his energetic
efforts contributed to the institutional development of the
medical faculty. Faculty and students increasingly sought
postgraduate training abroad, as the missionary model for
medical education shifted towards the development of Chinese professors of medicine who could carry out scientific
research and the expansion of medical education in Sichuan.

The goals of the College of Dentistry, which amalgamated
with the College of Medicine in 1929, were more consistently
focused on the education of a scientific elite. The founder and
dean of the school, Dr A.W. Lindsay, was committed to establishing a nationally recognized university-level training program in dentistry, whose graduates would promote dental
education and research in China. Lindsay also aspired to
advise Chinese governments on the development of a national
dental service. Until 1939 WCUU offered the only university-
level dental training in China, and the college drew students
from all over the country. It continues to be the leading dental institution in China to the present day.

The exigencies of China's wartime needs for medical service
disrupted this effort in the mid-1940s, as the Guomindang
conscripted, first, all graduates, and eventually all final-year
students, for military medical service. Government medical
schools were dedicated to fulfilling the national medical plan
to train doctors to serve the needs of a large population. During this time WCUU and the other Christian medical schools
were criticized for their elitist approach to medical education.
The members of the graduating class of 1944 were admon-
ished by Dr Hu Ding-an, an official of the National Health
Administration (NHA) in Chongqing, to revise their ambitions
to be more congruent with China's needs: 'You are an elite.
You are over-educated ... The future for those who indulge in
competitive specialization in urban centres is that you won't

make much of a contribution towards relieving the disease and suffering of the nation.'[58]

Despite the disruption of the war years, the college maintained its pursuit of academic excellence. In 1949, on the thirty-eighth anniversary of the founding of the university, the last president before the school's nationalization in 1950 addressed the graduating class. He reviewed the school's history of commitment to nurturing qualified students who were both capable of research and committed to society. However, the university's policy of elitist medical education and its failure to develop public health as an important sphere of medicine,[59] drew government criticism from both the Guomindang and, later, the Communists. Dr Li Ting-an contributed an article to the student medical journal in 1944 indicating that although the Soviet system of health care would not be adopted in China, their model of health-care delivery, which gave equal weight to curative and preventive medicine, was appropriate for China. This model formed the NHA's plan for the organization of 'medical benefits to all classes of society.'[60] When the missionaries introduced scientific medicine in Sichuan, there were no government plans for the administration of health care; medical care was not even remotely a concern of government. Now that the Chinese government controlled medical service and education, it had different priorities for these Western-trained medical graduates. In Chiang Kai-shek's plan for the postwar reconstruction of China, he emphasized the role of public health and set the goal of training 232,500 medical personnel within ten years after the war.[61] Until China's basic health needs could be met, the Guomindang government was content to let foreigners remain teaching in foreign-subsidized institutions, while their Chinese graduates administered medical services.

The university's response to changing conditions and expectations was reflected in policy shifts over a twenty-five year period. In 1925 it was acknowledged that the university's devolution to Chinese authority was slower than expected, 'with little in actual accomplishment up to the present time.'[62] The initial contribution of foreign faculty and foreign

funding was showing no signs of having outlived its usefulness. On the contrary, the institution continued to expand in
spite of increasing restraints on its finances by the postwar
depression in Canada and the United States. In 1933 the Laymen's Foreign Missions Inquiry identified the 'uneconomic
character of the university' to be due to the proliferation of
small departments and the vested interests of faculty in their
particular fields of study. The report rationalized this tendency in the medical field by arguing that the College of Medicine and Dentistry was the only institution providing medical
education in West China, and, furthermore, that its dental
training was likely the best available in all of China. The
university's vice-president, Dr G.S. Sparling, argued that devolution was severely hampered by the unavailability of
adequate Chinese staff and the difficulty in recruiting teachers
from other provinces to remote Sichuan.[63] The result was an
emphasis on recruiting foreign staff, both to bolster the department faculties and to hasten the training of Chinese replacements. The demand for highly qualified specialists for
the university, as opposed to general practitioners for station
hospitals,[64] reflected the increasing gap between overall
mission goals and those of the professional institution.

The organizational changes in 1929, whereby the medical
and dental colleges were amalgamated, and the clinical hospitals were united under a single hospitals board, were indicative of the increasing centralization of administration. The
'internal administration' of each unit was to remain autonomous, regarding finances and training, but policy formula-
tion was centralized. This was done to facilitate better use of
teaching resources for an increasing number of students,[65] a
strictly pragmatic consideration. Conflicting attitudes towards
the institutionalization of the university were evident in the
response to an attempt to finance a new teaching hospital for
the medical college. Dr Joseph Beech, chancellor of WCUU,
proposed selling the three outmoded mission hospitals in
Chengdu to pay for one new, modern hospital. While the
medical faculty were 'for the most part sympathetic to the
proposal,' most of the missionaries objected. Beech had of-

fered to sell the Canadian Si Sheng Ci Hospital to one of the Chengdu militarists as a municipal hospital, but the evangelical missionaries opposed the idea of giving up such a bastion of Christian influence. While the Mission Council in Chengdu could appreciate 'the need of the medical men' for a clinical hospital, they did not approve of sacrificing a distinctly mission (as opposed to university) hospital to finance it.[66]

The professional interests of the medical faculty were further demonstrated by Leslie Kilborn's demand for additional medical staff, particularly dental staff to maintain the reputation and prestige of the dental school.[67] In his response, Endicott chastised Kilborn for putting the clinical needs of the medical school above the evangelical goals of the mission. He pointed out that Kilborn's father, Omar Kilborn, had advocated the view that hospital work was primarily a tool of evangelism and that the board's decisions regarding allocation of personnel would be made on that basis.[68] At the same time, however, the Mission Secretary, Gerald Bell, and the chief of surgery at the university, Dr E.C. Wilford, were urging the appointment of a surgeon to the college, arguing that surgery made a special contribution towards the acceptance of modern medicine (and, by extension, to the acceptance of Christian influence).[69] Bell attributed the policy conflicts among the missionaries to their differing perceptions of mission goals. The younger professionals at the university stressed the broader goals of the Social Gospel and criticized the station evangelists for their own institutional emphasis on the building of a church.[70] Even the young professionals, however, questioned the increasing cost and scope of the university in the face of severe financial constraints. Dr Bruce Collier, the highly respected professor of biochemistry, suggested in 1934 that changing circumstances called for a review of policy: 'The financial situation has created great hardship in the carrying on of institutional work here, and one begins to wonder how far this type of work is justified ... It may be that a better policy would be to get out among the people, and work 'from the bottom up.'[71] Collier's response to the

institutionalization of the medical college's goals was not
typical of his colleagues, and he resigned in 1939, disillusioned with the direction the university was taking. The
more general division of attitudes was between the 'mission
group' and the 'university group,' who were in perpetual conflict over goals and, consequently, financial policy.[72] Limited
funds were available for mission medical work. The question
was, where could they be most effectively used to achieve the
essential goal of the mission, and what was that goal: social
change or evangelization?

The evacuation of the Guomindang government and universities to Sichuan in 1938 was a turning point in the development of the WCUU. Leslie Kilborn interpreted the implications
of this move for the university: 'Possibly one of the events of
greatest significance will be the whole-hearted realization that
China's centre of culture now lies in her Far West. With her
educational institutions and the bulk of her intellectual leadership concentrated in three Western provinces, we may look
forward to a place of increasingly great importance for the
West China Union University.'[73]

The university campus served as host to four refugee universities – Jinling, Nanjing, Qilu (Cheeloo, Shandong Christian
University), Yenjing (Yenching)[74] – and the PUMC School of
Nursing. The influx raised the number of students from four
hundred to a thousand in a six-month period.[75] These were
heady times for the previously isolated 'backwoods' campus,
and the missionaries envisioned that their influence on this
group of students would provide 'leaders destined to create
and shape a new China.'[76]

The increasing importance of Chengdu as a cultural centre
was accomplished by the development of Sichuan's Provincial
Health Administration and the location of the National
Health Administration in the province. The sophisticated
Chinese medical institutions and personnel from 'downriver'
(the coastal regions and industrial cities) stimulated the medical missionaries to meet their challenge by either competing
or cooperating. Both responses were apparent. Leslie Kilborn
suggested to the mission board that 'with government educa-

tion constantly improving ... with the necessity of maintaining higher and therefore costlier standards,' it might be advisable to amalgamate the two major Christian medical schools, Qilu and West China, to improve their efficiency and standards.[77] A new university hospital was finally realized, funded by the China Medical Board and the Guomindang government which used West China's facilities for their medical students. The institution was thus expanding, and Kilborn, seeing the role of the medical college as increasingly important, requested that the board provide a university school of nursing, an emergency department, and administrative staff, full plumbing and central heating, and additional medical staff.[78] Kilborn's frustrations of many years erupted under the stimulus of the better-staffed, better-equipped institutions from East China, which were liberal with their criticisms of West China's failings.[79]

Another response to the challenge of the more prestigious government universities was to refrain from competition and to concentrate on 'moral and character education.'[80] This suggestion came from Dr R.C. Spooner, professor of chemistry at the university, who felt that the university emphasized 'utilitarian aspects of the work as against other, equally vital phases of Christian university education.'[81] Spooner criticized the institutionalization of the university's goals, referring to the policy that led to the expansion of the university: 'if we have a good man, we immediately have to start a department.'[82] Spooner's recommendations were not in opposition to Kilborn's policy of concentrating mission efforts in one high quality institution. Both emphasized the goal of developing medical leadership. Spooner, however, emphasized moral education, while Kilborn stressed professional education. It was generally agreed, however, that mission policy should concentrate on the medical schools as the cornerstone of medical missionary endeavour.[83]

Paradoxically, the expansion of the medical college led to its decline. Maintaining the university hospital as a modern teaching institution was far more costly than maintaining the mission hospitals.[84] In 1945 eleven members of the medical faculty left Chengdu, with no replacements, and the teaching hospitals were operating on a serious deficit.[85] The medical school had relied on teaching staff from the refugee universities, and when they departed in 1946, the remaining staff was inadequate to carry on.[86] In spite of this crisis in funding and staff, Kilborn continued to envision the growth of the institution; he requested a grant from the China Medical Board for the establishment of a child guidance clinic to aid in the training of medical students.[87] The grant request was denied in view of the urgency of maintaining the already existing work.[88]

The missionaries who remained were exhausted by the war and felt abandoned by the home mission board, which was not sending replacements to maintain an adequate staff.[89] Postwar inflation in China, combined with the reduction in staff, contributed to the further deterioration of the College of Medicine and Dentristy. Kilborn, however, maintained his optimism and determination to keep the college going and to increase its effectiveness.[90] He proposed that the United Church take full responsibility for the university staff, arguing that it was already a Canadian institution: 'without the Canadian personnel this would become a non-missionary institution ... It would be taken over by the government within a few years.'[91] This was both the irony and the core of the medical missionaries' dilemma: At what point did they devolve the medical work to the Chinese? What combination of professional competence, Christian values, and Christian commitment determined the achievement of their goal?

Devolution of the College of Medicine and Dentistry

The pessimistic attitude of the medical missionaries towards devolution of responsibility to their Chinese colleagues, especially prior to the influx of 'downriver' doctors in 1938, may have been due to Sichuan's remoteness and minimal exposure to the influence of Western education. Dr Gladys Cunningham, who studied at PUMC during 1927–9, when the anti-Christian riots forced the evacuation of foreigners from

Chengdu, was surprised at the ability of the Chinese staff at that institute, and changed her attitude to the future of devolution: '... it was also a very good thing for us to see Chinese doing medical work so well as many of them do it. It gave us a most cheering slant on them and many a time in the future when we are discouraged with our material, it will help us to keep going and striving towards that which we have seen is possible – i.e. *Chinese doing scientific medicine in a scientific way.*'[92] However, the disorganization of the mission medical work on the return of the missionaries to Sichuan in 1929 was disheartening. Missionaries were hesitant to dismiss inefficient, incompetent staff for fear of anti-Christian reprisals.[93]

By 1931, however, Leslie Kilborn reported with great enthusiasm that two WCUU graduates had established a successful municipal hospital at Hanzhou, near Chengdu, and enlisted the talents of two more graduates the following year. Although he pointed out that an increase in non-mission hospitals would create competition with the mission, he was optimistic about the development of hospitals 'under Chinese management.'[94]

Within the university, it was generally agreed that devolution was a long way off. Bruce Collier, the professor of biochemistry, indicated that the backwardness of Sichuan, compared with the 'downriver universities,' clouded the prospects for 'building up a permanent Chinese staff.'[95] Ashley Lindsay also remarked on the low level of pre-university education in Sichuan, the scarcity of second-generation Christians in Sichuan compared with East China, and, therefore, the scarcity of suitable candidates for faculty appointments.[96] C.C. Chen, provincial commissioner of health for Sichuan and a PUMC graduate, attributed the lack of devolution to the University's backward administration. He expressed the opinion that the school did not meet China's needs, and that a 'mere missionary institution' had little hope of contributing to China's reconstruction unless it was made a provincial institution.[97] A critique of the WCUU faculty was delivered by Dean C.W. Chang of the Nanjing University, department of agriculture, who accused the faculty of refusing 'to acknowledge their academic incompetence [sic],' and of having an 'unconscious policy of foreign superiority and keeping Chinese subordinate.'[98] The mistrust was mutual; the Chinese thought the WCUU faculty was sub-standard, and the missionaries feared giving control of their institution to incompetent Chinese, particularly those who were not Christian.[99] The wife of a leading faculty member criticized the vested interests of senior missionary faculty as the stumbling block to devolution.[100] Her husband acknowledged that, after twenty years, the Chinese staff were ready to take over undergraduate teaching, leaving the missionary medical staff free for advanced teaching. He stated: 'I am not one of those who turn responsibility over to the Chinese staff before they are at all capable of taking it.'[101]

The missionaries were concerned with the prestige of the medical college and wanted to maintain high standards in order to exert maximum influence. They were therefore reluctant to relinquish control of the institution. Furthermore, the university was responsible to the mission as a whole, and many WCUU graduates were appointed to staff the station hospitals, and their opportunities for postgraduate training and future university positions thereby restricted. There were some subtle, and some blatant, indications of foreign arrogance towards Chinese colleagues. For example, in 1943, missionary residences stood empty while Chinese faculty were crowded into decrepit temporary accommodations on campus.[102] Dr Claude E. Forkner of PUMC related the assessment of other missionary groups that 'the Chengtu missionaries are twenty years behind the times.' Forkner wrote that he thought 'the attitude of some of the missionaries was definitely wrong,' and that eventually the government would nationalize educational institutions and eliminate foreign administration.[103] There were those who argued that the university should be under the authority of the indigenous Chinese church. Others maintained that the Chinese faculty, even though they were Christians, were not ready to take over positions of authority in the departments. The Chinese church was a small and relatively powerless institution and could never hope to undertake the financial support of a modern medical school. As late as 1946 one senior evangelical missionary suggested it was time to start the process of devolution, but that the medical work must be 'made a permanent part of the Christian movement in China' under church administration.[104]

By the time Chinese physicians were given leadership positions in the university, it was embarrassingly late. By 1947 Dr Clifford Tsao (Cao Zhongliang) was appointed dean of medicine, Dr Y.T. Beh (Bai Yingcai) was superintendant of the university hospital, and Dr T.H. Lan (Lan Tianhe) was head of biochemistry.[105] In 1950 Dr Gladys Cunningham gave up the chair in obstetrics and gynecology to her student Dr Helen Yoh (Yue Yichen).[106] On 1 January 1951 the university was taken over by the Chinese Communists,[107] and devolution was no longer an issue, except as an issue in the campaign against Christian cultural aggression.[108]

In assessing the extent to which the medical missionaries at the university devolved authority to the Chinese, it is argued that their apparent failure in this respect did not signify their failure to achieve their goals. As a result of the vested interests of senior professors in their individual departments, of the ever-expanding scope of the institution, and of the consequent confusion of institutional goals with mission goals, the medical missionaries were reluctant to divest themselves of the authority to administer what they perceived as their institution. Furthermore, there were no circumscribed standards to indicate at what point they had achieved their objectives. Had a medical missionary in 1920 been told that by 1938 Sichuan would have its own Provincial Health Administration, and municipal hospitals, *xian* health stations and a government medical school with Western-trained faculty, he might have said that the medical missionaries had outlived their usefulness and that it was time to go home. However, a medical missionary in 1940 would measure China's medical modernization by different standards. True, the government had an elaborate health administration, and medical schools, but officials could not possibly achieve their goals of providing health care for China's vast population without external assistance. Moreover, China's medical profession was not predominantly Christian, nor was its population, and there was still the opportunity to exert Christian influence. The gauge for 'the best of modern medicine' had changed dramatically since 1888, and it continued to change as medical science and technology advanced. And the measure of 'Christian values' was at best ephemeral. What the missionaries did accomplish, however, was the establishment in Sichuan of an institute for modern medical education, the mobilization of social and political elites to participate in the development of health care and medical education, and the formation of a professional technological elite upon which to build an indigenous health-care system. In the process, they also served as a valuable resource to the administrators who were developing China's health services.

University-Government Relations

This section examines two aspects of the medical missionaries' relationship to Chinese government attempts to modernize health care. The first aspect of the relationship is the missionaries' efforts to devolve financial responsibility to the Chinese government for health-care development. The second involves the changing relationship between the missionaries and government, from agents, advisers, and teachers, to subordinates, albeit essential ones, to the Chinese administration.

As early as 1925, when Sichuan's government was characterized as much by its absence as by its unreliability, Joseph Beech, WCUU's president, encouraged Governor-General Yang Sen (who controlled Chengdu at the time) to participate with the university in the development of medical education and services for the province. Beech indicated that the university personnel 'have always enjoyed the most intimate relations with the government authorities here.'[109] Recognizing that the government did not have the revenue to contribute to such a project, he requested a grant on Yang Sen's behalf from the

American Boxer Indemnity Fund.[110] This effort was designed in part to secure indirectly, for the medical school, funds not readily available to a Christian institution. Primarily it was a plan to integrate the university's work in health-care development with local political forces.

A further move to involve government with the university, at least by way of recognition, was the immediate compliance with the national government mandate for the registration of private schools and hospitals, issued in August of 1927. By September of that year, the Provincial Educational Bureau in Sichuan had not been officially informed of this regulation, and asked Dr Beech: 'with whom do you wish to register, the Nanking Government, the Northern Government, or the Hankow Government?'[111] The missionaries, in spite of the obvious political instability of China, submitted their application for registration as a gesture of faith in the local government, and in order to protect the institution in case of future regulations.[112] The regulations for hospital registration were a clear indication of the Nanjing government's attempt to use mission institutions as a basis for their health-care delivery system. The regulations demanded that hospitals be under the jurisdiction of the health department and that they appoint a Chinese superintendant, provide hospital care for the poor, and serve as health centres. Dr H.S. Houghton of the Peking Union Medical College reported that 'this control is largely nominal to give face to the Health Department.'[113] However, it was a recognition by the Nationalist government that provision of a health-care system was a function of government and that missionary institutions were a valuable resource which could lend credibility to the government's health program. In 1933, the WCUU registered with the Nationalist government at Nanjing,[114] and in 1934, the first 'practical recognition of the work being done by the University was shown by a grant of $20,000 in silver by the Nanking Government.'[115] Generalissimo and Madame Chiang Kai-shek were particularly interested in the university, whose agriculture department supplied them with dairy products and fresh produce.[116] The government gave funds for a chair in the College of Dentistry in 1935;[117] and it was said that Dr H.J. Mullett, who provided Chiang with dentures, 'put the teeth into the Japanese resistance.'[118]

In the absence of their own infrastructure for the administration of health care services, the National Health Administration's (NHA) epidemic prevention bureau distributed vaccines and serums through the pathology department of the College of Medicine, under Dr T.H. Williams. In addition, Williams's laboratory provided a diagnostic service for the hospitals in West China.[119]

The dental college in particular was recognized by the NHA for its leadership. A.W. Lindsay served as an adviser on the NHA's dental committee, which endeavoured to create 'a national programme for dental teaching, the nucleus for which is our Dental College.'[120] In 1949 Lindsay's former students, the National Dental Board of Health, and the West China Dental Association honoured him as 'the founder of scientific dentistry in China.'[121] The Chinese ambassador to Canada, Liu Jie, communicated to the Canadian Department of External Affairs that Lindsay would be awarded the Order of the Auspicious Star of the Republic of China[122] for his pioneering contribution in 'the promotion of dental studies in China and ... in raising the standard of dental health throughout the country.'[123] Dr W. Crawford, professor of public health at the university, was also offered this official recognition, for his contributions 'to the field of medicine ... and especially in view of his medical services in China during World War II.'[124]

The medical missionaries played a distinctive role in the development of Sichuan's Provincial Health Administration (PHA). Leslie Kilborn expressed his interest in 1938 in cooperating with a provincial health service when one came into existence.[125] In May 1939 Dr C.C. Chen was appointed director of the first Sichuan Provincial Health Administration, as a result of the provincial government's recognition of 'the importance of public health.' Chen stressed 'close cooperation with the mission hospitals' as a 'means of helping the people,' and entered into cooperation with the university's department of pharmacology to manufacture common drugs and medical supplies.[126] The WCUU participated in the Sichuan Public Health Training Institute, which provided personnel for the administration's health centres.[127] The United Hospital of the Canadian mission supplied laboratory facilities for the training of laboratory technologists for the government's Institute of Infectious Diseases.[128] Although Dr Chen remarked that the WCUU medical college was inadequate and 'knew nothing of the needs of the health system in China,'[129] the faculty made a significant contribution to the development of government resources for health administration.

The development of national capabilities for health-care delivery resulted in a shift in the relationship between the Guomindang government and medical missionaries. Whereas previously the government had been dependent on missionary facilities and resources, after 1941 it began consciously to view mission medical work as instrumental to national needs. In 1941 the mission was alarmed that the PHA was setting up *xian* health centres and competing with the mission for medical personnel.[130] Guomindang policy was to choose strategic locations for their health-service centres, disregarding the existence of mission hospitals, and thus competing with them for patients.[131] Chen's perspective was that the standards of missionary hospitals were not high, and that they stressed curative rather than preventive medicine.[132] The missionaries were gradually being replaced by an indigenous force for medical care, and they reacted cautiously to this threat to their sovereignty.

In 1944 the National Health Administration requested cooperation from Christian hospitals in their plan for China's postwar rehabilitation, but emphasized the subordinate role of Christian medical work.[133] The NHA expected mission hospitals 'to function within the framework of the Government Health Service, of which they will have to form a part.' This would place the university under the authority of both the minister of health and the minister of education, to whose regulations they had to conform.[134] The Nationalist government, although it did not have the resources to carry out its full program for public health, was now in full control of the administration of health services.

In 1951 the Communist government requested the services of three of the Canadian medical missionaries to continue teaching at the nationalized West China University. The missionaries could not accept the tightening controls on religious and academic freedom, and one medical missionary in Chongqing was imprisoned by the Communists on a charge of refusing to turn over mission drug supplies to the authorities.[135] On 4 January 1951, the board closed the West China Mission and instructed the missionaries to return to Canada.[136]

Summary and Conclusion

The West China Union University College of Medicine and Dentistry was founded to train leaders of China's medical modernization; its goal was eventually to devolve the institution to Chinese authority. It therefore adopted an elitist model of medical education, with seven years of training in basic sciences and clinical skills. Faced with the tremendous local needs for medical service, the medical faculty decided it could make its most effective contribution by concentrating its limited resources on medical education. Although the institution did not achieve a reputation for excellence in scientific teaching, it did serve as a valuable resource for the development of China's, and particularly Sichuan's, health-care system.

The college laboured under the constraints of inadequate funding and personnel and further suffered from the academic isolation of Sichuan from the rest of China and from Western intellectual influence. Preclinical instruction of students had to compensate for their relatively low level of secondary education, and teaching in Chinese was cumbersome and strenuous for Canadian faculty, who had to master a difficult language, one which did not have an equivalent vocabulary for scientific terminology. In spite of its policy of concentration on educational goals, the college was faced with the demand for staffing of its affiliated mission hospitals, to compensate for the shortage of missionary personnel. Because the college functioned as both a service institution and a teaching institution, its staff and budget were stressed to the limit. There was no time or money provided for research, and thus the college did not develop as a scientific institution. Unlike PUMC, which was the model for an elite educational centre in the medical field, WCUU did not attract accomplished researchers and had limited funds to provide post-graduate fellowships abroad for its students. In the early years, the college did not have an administrative staff, and its professors were burdened with excessive paperwork in addition to their teaching and clinical responsibilities.

Despite these disadvantages, the medical work expanded, and its growth surpassed that of the Chinese church and evangelical missions. Its goals became autonomous, distinct from those of the mission, and as the institution became differentiated, its objectives were increasingly secularized. What was initially an evangelical mission to the Chinese became a source of advisory, material, and technical assistance to Chinese government efforts towards the development of a health-care system.

The medical missionaries failed to devolve the administration of their own institution to their Chinese colleagues. This may be explained by the gradual institutionalization of the goals of the college, which conflicted with mission goals for Christianization of the medical profession as a means of evangelizing the nation, rather than as an end in itself. The confusion of these goals was one of the factors that inhibited the missionaries from relinquishing control of the institution. Another major factor was the 'empire building' tendency of senior faculty members, who had vested interests in preserving the achievements of a lifetime of work and who were unwilling to risk the school's deterioration in the hands of junior faculty members.

The greatest obstacle to devolution, however, was the cost of maintaining a modern medical institution. The teaching hospital, which also provided free medical services, was not a source of remuneration, but an excessive financial burden to the medical school and mission. The lengthy curriculum, designed to train teachers, was costly and extravagant in the face of the desperate need for medical services and the financial constraints of the mission. Had there been no concurrent development of China's medical system, with its own priorities for personnel and institutional development, the College of Medicine might have been viewed more favorably as establishing the foundation for medical care. However, the policy of the university did not adapt to changing conditions, either in China or in its own institution and constituency of support. It could not maintain the scope it had established prior to 1927, and rather than retrench the mission attempted to spread its meagre resources to cover medical education and medical service in the station hospitals. The institution thus deteriorated to the point of having a minimum of staff and equipment with which to carry on medical education.

When the missionaries left China in 1951, however, they left the medical school in the charge of doctors whom they had trained and financed for postgraduate study in Canada. The medical college was renamed Sichuan Medical College in 1952, and several of these alumni held leading positions on its staff. In terms of contributing a corps of medical professionals to China, the missionaries succeeded in the 'multiplication of ourselves.'

4

Evangelists of Science:
The Medical Missionaries

The expressed goal of the professional medical missionaries in Sichuan Province was the 'multiplication of ourselves:' They sought to train highly skilled medical professionals, like themselves, imbued with the principles of Western scientific learning and the Christian ethics of service and humanitarianism. Furthermore, they were part of an international movement of evangelization, first promulgated by the American Student Volunteer Movement and later the Student Christian Movement. To explore further the factors which informed their perceptions and goals, this chapter provides a profile of the medical missionary. It examines the ideal attributes of the medical missionary, recruitment patterns from 1891 to 1949, term of service, geographic origins of medical missionaries, their socioeconomic background and educational background, the motivations of the medical missionary volunteers, and the ideology of Canadian medical professionals during the first half of the twentieth century.

A Profile of the Medical Missionaries

The Ideal Medical Missionary

Missionary volunteers were recruited by the General Board of Missions of the Methodist Church prior to 1925 and by the Board of Foreign Missions of the United Church of Canada after church union in 1925.[1] Although medical policy was decided in the field by the mission council and its medical committee, the board in Toronto was responsible for screening and appointing medical personnel.[2] An analysis of their concept of the ideal medical missionary, and how that concept changed over time, provides a useful indicator of whom they attempted to recruit to medical missionary service.

Over half the Canadian medical personnel in Sichuan were recruited before church union in 1925. Of the sixty medical missionaries recruited between 1891 and 1952, forty-five sailed for China before 1925, and of these, seventeen continued to serve after 1925. The first doctors to enter the mission field did so during a time when, in most mission fields, medical work was a minor adjunct to evangelical work, a means of attracting reluctant converts, winning their confidence, and thus opening the door for the message of the Gospel.[3] In many cases it was simply the Christian response of the evangelical missionary to relieve suffering. Medical work was little more than first aid, and medical training was correspondingly limited.[4] The concept of sending fully trained doctors as missionaries was unorthodox, and it had to be introduced gently. Thus, Omar Kilborn's appeal for medical missionaries in 1910, and his description of the ideal candidate, were carefully couched in acceptable terms: 'Nowadays the medical man is regarded as a *Medical missionary*. Not only must his moral character be above reproach ... but he must be a positive type of consecrated missionary, thoroughly evangelistic in tone and aim ...'[5] In contradiction to this insistence that evangelical goals were the primary motivation, Kilborn went on to describe the ideal medical missionary as a highly trained professional who ought not to waste time in theological training.[6] Kilborn also introduced the criteria of mental health and social adaptability, in addition to the requirement of physical fitness, to ensure that the medical missionary recruit would be a sound investment for the mission board of the church. This emphasis would appeal to the lay businessmen who were gradually taking over the administration of the mission field in the early 1900s and applying the rational ideals of pragmatism and efficiency to achieve the goal of 'World Evangelization in This Generation.'[7] Besides being motivated by the 'joy of service' and the 'beauty of sacrifice,' the medical missionary was to possess the 'vision splendid' of a 'great nation which has been permeated and rejuvenated by the Christian ideals of justice and purity, of love and service.'[8]

By the early 1920s it was no longer necessary to apologize for the medical aspect of missionary work. In *Medical Missions: The Twofold Task*, Walter Lambuth, one of the earliest American medical missionaries and an assistant editor of the Peking-based *Medical Missionary Journal*,[9] described the ideal medical missionary as a dedicated professional whose task was 'to bridge the chasm between the religious and the secular,' by applying the scientific spirit to solve the needs of 'the body and the soul of man.'[10] Lambuth, like Kilborn ten years earlier, stressed physical and mental health as essential qualifications of a candidate, as well as 'spiritual conviction' and 'fine character,' in that order.[11] The argument for stressing strong moral and physical character and high educational standards was justified by the high cost of supporting medical missionaries. One contemporary analyst suggests that in lieu of an 'economical probationary system,' this was 'the safest policy' to protect the mission board's investment. The medical missionary, he proposes, was harder to replace than an evangelist, nurse, or schoolteacher.[12] As for motivation, the tone of Lambuth's appeal was not greatly different from those which had been heard since the late nineteenth century: not as outspokenly arrogant, he nevertheless alluded to the opportunity open to young Christians to 'save the lost,' 'to restore shrunken capacity,' or in other words, to bring the heathen nations up to the standards of the Christian nations. The medical missionary's relation to the natives was 'that of a brother in sympathy, and of a father in counsel.'[13]

Prior to 1925 the increasing importance of professional qualifications characterized the change in expectations of the medical missionary; the basic motivation of evangelization, however, remained constant. The year of church union, 1925,

marked a turning point in this identification of missionary
medical work as an exclusive province of evangelism. Chapter
1 discusses the changes in church policy, with the increasing
emphasis on the secular aspects of the Social Gospel. Great
changes were also occurring in the mission field. The May
Fourth Movement in 1919 had galvanized Chinese student
nationalism to reject Western imperialism and to view it as
the root cause of China's political and economic weakness.[14]
From 1922 to 1925, this rising nationalism was manifested in
the anti-Christian movement,[15] which culminated in the
evacuation of foreign missionaries from China's interior as
anti-foreign hostility escalated into violence.[16] This forced
missionaries to respond to, or at least to reconsider, Chinese
demands for devolution of authority, and a corresponding
change in Western attitudes of cultural superiority, including
the relinquishment of extraterritorial privileges.

The emphasis on the physical plant by the Board of Foreign
Missions had already identified Christian goals with material
progress. By 1920 it was clearly accepted that science and
Christianity were allies, as illustrated by an appeal for medical mission support: 'Insanitary hospitals are a reproach to
Western medical science and to Christianity.'[17] A group of
evacuated missionaries held a conference in 1927 to discuss
the 'Next Step in Devolution' as a response to Chinese
demands, and they decided to facilitate devolution by first
devolving the authority of the mission council to separate
departmental boards. Thus, medical work was administrative-
ly separated from evangelical work. Dr A.S. Allen, representative of the medical missionaries at the conference, stressed
the primacy of developing Chinese medical professionals to
work in the movement to devolve 'modern hospitals and
modern medicine' to Chinese control.[18]

The 1936 United Church of Canada 'Report of the Special
Committee on Policy (Medical Work)' responded to this separation of church and hospital by recognizing that although
scientific medicine had been introduced in China by Christian
missions, and had developed independently of governments
and local community control, the time had come to integrate,

albeit selectively, with government and community health activities. The identification of science with Christianity, in the minds of these policy-makers, now appeared complete: 'If the ancestral faith in magic is destroyed by conversion to Christianity, it must be replaced by scientific medicine.'[19]

By the time the International Missionary Council met at Madras in 1938, the ideal medical missionary had evolved into a more obvious agent of secular modernization. While the recruitment standards still stressed religious conviction and fine moral character, the foremost requirement was 'the best possible professional qualifications.' In addition to these qualifications, the conference members were cognizant of the demands of rising nationalism in the countries of the mission fields; they were not unaware of the secular forces competing with the church to serve the needs of the rural poor, and they stressed their commitment to cooperate with, but never compete with, non-Christian health work. Sensitive to accusations of imperialistic motives, especially of the earlier generation of missionaries who grew up with the belief in the 'white man's burden' to civilize the heathen nations, and whose presence in China was under the protection of the foreign powers' gunboats, these missionaries recognized the need to identify mission goals with the needs of the nations in which they served. The modern medical missionary was required to be free of a sense of racial superiority and to make every effort 'to foster friendly co-operation with local practitioners, and with governments and communities that are promoting health programmes.'[20]

In the International Missionary Council document, the 'heathen' nations were referred to less offensively as the 'unevangelized'; the medical missionary's role became less that of a messenger of God and more that of an agent of social reconstruction. The missionary's goal, as expressed in the 1936 United Church policy statement, was to foster understanding between races, classes, and nations and thus contribute to political stability, to 'ordered society.'[21]

By the time the McGill neurosurgeon Wilder Penfield was sent by the National Research Council of Canada to report on medical work in 'Free China,'[22] the secular evolution of the medical missionary was complete. Missionaries were no longer being actively recruited; China's political instability during the Sino-Japanese War made the future of the Chinese missions too uncertain. However, the mission board, impoverished by the cumulative demands of the economic depression of the 1930s, followed by the Second World War and rampant inflation in China, hoped to continue to develop its financial investment in the medical mission plant and sought government approval and funding for its work.[23] The medical missionaries, who wanted to contribute to China's postwar reconstruction, now needed the approbation of both their own government and the Chinese government, as the cost of a modern medical school and hospital was beyond the means of a private institution. Penfield observed that the Christian missions arrived in China 'before the process of Westernization began. They have given the Chinese people the best example our civilization could produce – considerably better than we deserve!' He attested to the fact that 'these medical missionaries have become educators ... They do not proselyte. They are too busy healing the sick. They train Chinese doctors and plan to step aside in favour of the Chinese as soon as suitable men are trained.'[24] The figure Penfield described in 1943 was a long stride from the itinerant evangelist who dispensed first aid.

The development of the foreign mission board's application for medical missionaries illustrates the changes in the notion of the ideal medical missionary during the half century from 1891 to 1941. The earliest extant application form is dated 1898. Presumably the first medical missionaries set up this relatively systematic method of screening applicants once they had surveyed the needs of the mission field. The form consisted of one page, half of which contained a printed oath attesting to the fact that the applicant had been 'truly converted to God and ... called by the Holy Spirit to go as a missionary to the heathen.'[25] The form asked whether the applicant was applying for medical or evangelistic work, and specified that the term of service was for life. The minimal information required in the half page of questions included condition of health, education, references, indebtedness, previous occupation, and marital status. An example of the terseness of the application was Dr W.J. Sheridan's reply in 1906 to the question about the condition of his health: 'Good.'[26] By 1907 the form included several more specific questions about educational background and choice of field, but there was no change in format until 1921. The religious requirement of the 'conversion experience' was maintained, as was the reference to the 'heathen.' By this date, however, the mission plant had expanded in size and complexity, and the type of worker was now left blank. No longer were the recruits classed as medical or evangelical; there were now builders, printers, dentists, accountants, and a variety of professionals needed to run a burgeoning institution.

The application form for 1931 reflected a growing concern with the contractual arrangement between missionaries and the Board of Foreign Missions and with the motivation and health of the applicant. The revised form stated a preference for volunteers less than thirty years of age to facilitate the learning of a new language. Where one question about the condition of health had satisfied the board previously, there were now ten, dealing with mental health, personality traits, and habits, as well as physical stamina. The applicant's theological convictions were examined not by an oath swearing to the divine call, but by seven questions covering motivations, theological knowledge, and personal religious experience. The available applications indicate that candidates' responses were brief and demonstrated a knowledge of basic Christian theology. Although one candidate chose to disregard the questions with the explanation: 'This is presumably for clerical candidates,' the others made a serious attempt to answer questions about what their 'message' would be:

As to the Bible;
As to the World and its need;

As to the Person of Jesus Christ;
As to the life and death of Jesus Christ;
As to the Holy Spirit.

This attempt to determine the lay missionary's evangelical
motivation was at least a formal statement that secular attributes were not the only criteria for appointment to the field.
The post-1921 applications were designed to recruit individuals who were both professionally and religiously qualified:
'Applicants must satisfy the Board as to missionary zeal, Bibli-
cal knowledge, aptitude to teach, ability to acquire the language of the people to whom they may be sent, and as to their
equipment for the department of work for which they seek
appointment.'[27]

In summary, changes in the application form show an increasing concern for professional qualifications and physical
and mental health, reflecting the criteria for selecting medical
missionaries which Omar Kilborn had suggested in 1910.[28]
The growth of psychiatry and psychology as legitimate fields
of study no doubt contributed to the mission board's increasing concern with the mental and emotional soundness of
prospective missionaries. By 1940 it was even suggested that
the requisite medical examinations for physical fitness should
be supplemented by a psychiatric evaluation.[29] This interest
in the medical missionary's health status reflected the board's
recognition that the life of a foreign medical missionary was
stressful, because of the inherent demands of huge numbers
of patients and inadequate facilities and the political instability frequently manifested in anti-foreign hostility.

Another perspective on the ideal medical missionary can be
gained from an analysis of letters of reference attached to the
missionary application forms. These letters give us an idea
not only of what the missionaries were like, but of what their
referees thought were the most important attributes of medical missionaries. An analysis of the content of these letters
pertaining to thirty-two male applicants reveals that the
overwhelmingly important characteristics of the successful
candidate were amiability and adaptability. Of a total of 185
descriptive words used, ninety-nine referred to personality

traits, and eighty-nine of these were positive references. The profile which emerges is that of a group of men who were calm, cheerful, kind, devoted, genial, co-operative, popular, 'all round,' well-liked, and respected.

Second in importance was their intellectual ability, and only four of the thirty-two applicants in this group were described as below average in intellectual attainments and professional competence. The overall picture was that of a group of 'first-class students,' conscientious, of good judgment, initiative, and above-average intelligence.

Christian dedication was rated third in importance in terms of the frequency with which it was referred to. Only two of the candidates were perceived as having questionable motivations, with one described as having a 'temperament not suited to conversion,' and the other as being candidly secular in his intent. The majority were portrayed as 'sincere Christian gentlemen,' spiritually sound, with high moral character. Only one was described as a strong evangelist. Of the thirty-two applicants, seven were recommended for their physical strength. The rigours of mission work, especially in the remote reaches of West China, demanded men and women who were healthy and strong, and this group in particular was noted for 'splendid physique,' excellent health, physical fitness, and athletic prowess.

Recruitment: The Volunteers

In spite of the hardships of medical missionary life, there was a small (sixty in total) but steady stream of volunteers between 1891 and 1949. The years 1907 to 1910 saw the largest number of medical recruits since the establishment of the medical missions in the 1890s. During this three-year period, twelve new recruits sailed for China. This was followed by the postwar boom from 1917 to 1923,[30] when thirteen medical missionaries were posted to Sichuan. The earlier increase in volunteers might be explained by the influence of the youth-oriented Epworth League organized by Newton Rowell in 1887. This league, under the direction of F.C. Ste-

phenson, developed into a recruiting agency for foreign
missions, and was reorganized first into the Young People's
Forward Movement (1895) and later the Missionary Education
Movement (1908). Having grown up under the influence of
missionary activism as a goal of the church, students would
have been ready for the mission field at the time of the first
increase in recruitment. They had been exposed to the study
of social conditions, international politics, and the role of
education and public health in social amelioration, and many
had developed a strong 'missionary consciousness.' The postwar increase in recruits had a more obvious origin; thousands
of young soldiers were returning from the battlegrounds of
Europe. Many were reluctant to return to the prosaic life of
rural Canada, and they flocked to the cities for educational
and employment opportunities. The pattern of recruitment
also reflected political events in China. From 1924 to 1927,
only one medical missionary sailed for China. This was the
height of the anti-Christian movement, and most of the Sichuan missionaries were evacuated to the foreign concessions
of Shanghai by 1927. During the Nationalist Decade, however,
when the Guomindang government seemed poised to lead
China into modernity, thirteen medical missionaries joined
the West China Mission, to be part of China's revitalization.
This burst of activity was followed by a final slump in recruitment, which occurred after the outbreak of war in 1939. Most
of China was occupied by Japan, and transportation to China
was both scarce and hazardous. Furthermore, young Canadians in medical school were enlisting in their own military
forces. With the defeat of Japan in 1945 came the civil war in
China, culminating in the communist victory and eventual
expulsion of foreign missionaries.

    In the early years of medical mission development, the
Student Volunteer Movement (SVM) played an active role in
sensitizing university students to the needs of missions, and
the appeal to medical students was particularly effective. A
study of the SVM reports that of 8,140 volunteers recruited by
the movement between 1886 and 1919, 2,524 sailed for China.
Moreover, the Intercollegiate Missionary Alliance of Canada

amalgamated with SVM, and 'delegates from medical schools regularly attended the SVM conventions,' with a medical representative on the 'executive committee from 1898 onward.'[31] This study further points out the link between the China field and SVM recruits, suggesting that this educated elite of North America identified with the literati of China. The SVM students were challenged 'to convert these men of influence in China, and turn their influence unto the evangelization of their fellow-countrymen.'[32] Here was the embryo of the 'multiplication of ourselves' slogan.

As the SVM grew in North America, with the slogan 'World Evangelization In Our Time!' an increasing number of university students became involved in the missionary venture as an alternative to a career in Canada. There were many reasons motivating young graduates to seek work in the mission field, among them sincere dedication to the promotion of Christianity. Others sought adventure in exotic places, but as more graduates were trained in the rapidly expanding fields of science and technology, they sought to bring the benefits of their scientific education to countries where modernization was still an unknown process.

These young scientists, who became active in the Student Christian Movement (SCM), which grew out of the SVM, found in the missionary enterprise an avenue to introduce their ideas and technology to the non-Christian nations. Through medical missionary work, they exemplified the life of Christ by healing the sick, without directly preaching the Gospel. Perhaps more appealing to young professionals was the opportunity to pursue their careers where they were desperately needed and where they were afforded the prestige reserved for senior physicians at home. New medical graduates could expect to be directors of hospitals or clinics in rural China, while their counterparts in urban Canada would be struggling to establish themselves in a competitive market.

This alternative became even more appealing during the depression of the 1930s, when physicians could not always rely on reimbursement for services rendered. While missionary salaries were far from generous, they were reliable in a

time of great economic uncertainty. Thus, the inducements
of adventure, challenge, economic security, and, most important, the sense of moral obligation to serve the poor and the
suffering and to lead the developing nations on the path of
scientific progress motivated young medical students to serve
in the foreign mission field.

Term of Service

The number of missionaries in the field at any given time
fluctuated, with the interruptions of furloughs, leaves of
absence, local political upheavals, death, and disease. However, an examination of terms of service gives us an indication
of how many recruits left their mission field prematurely, that
is, before the 'service for life' period was up (see table 1).[33] Of
the forty-eight male medical missionaries (including thirty-
nine doctors, six dentists, two pharmacists, and one biochemist), seventeen stayed more than twenty-one years, nine
stayed from eleven to twenty years, and twenty-one stayed
ten years or less. A closer examination of the last group tells
us why so many of this group left. Of the twenty-one, the
service of six was terminated because of death or illness, three
resigned for unknown reasons, and two were disillusioned
with the work of the mission. Nine missionaries resigned
immediately following a political upheaval in China, and
three of these were expelled by the Communists after 1949.

The women medical missionaries are considered separately,
because they present a different pattern than the men. Of
thirteen recruits, five stayed more than twenty-one years, one
served from eleven to twenty years, and seven served ten
years or less. Of these seven, four retired when they married,
one when she had a child, one because of illness, and one
because of family responsibilities. If these seven are compared
to the six who continued full-time medical careers, marriage
and childbearing are not the obvious determinants of their
early retirement. Of these six full-time doctors, five were
married and two had children. It is postulated, however, that
the marriage partner had a significant influence. The husbands

TABLE 1
Term of service of medical missionaries

Term in years	1–10	11–20	21–40	
Men	21	9	17	(47)
Women	7	1	5	(13)
Total	28	10	22	60

of all five women were doctors themselves; and two were married to the same man (in succession). It is indicative of the expectations of woman recruits that a list of medical missionaries compiled in 1945 added the word 'Married' to the Retired/Deceased column for women medical missionaries.[34]

In sum, slightly over fifty per cent of the medical missionaries stayed longer than ten years in the field, or a significant portion of their active careers. Those who left early did so as a reaction to the strenuous demands of mission work, both physical and emotional.

Geographic Origins

The geographic influence of the Methodist Church, subsequently the United Church of Canada, and the demographic characteristics of Canada gave rise to a predominantly Ontario-born group of medical missionaries (see table 2). The Methodist Church and later United Church represented the largest Protestant denomination in the country. In the nation as a whole their membership accounted for an average of 17.5 per cent of the population, concentrated mainly in southern Ontario.[35] More than half of the medical missionaries were born in southern Ontario towns and cities (thirty-four out of sixty),[36] where Methodist and later United Church influence was strongest. Canada's domestic growth, from the time the first West China missionaries were recruited in 1891 to the closing of the mission in 1952, can be measured by a rapid increase in population and urbanization. From 1891 to 1950, Canada's population tripled, from 4,833,239 to 13,712,000. The population of Ontario, the home of the Methodist Church and

TABLE 2
Geographic origins of medical missionaries

Birthplace	Women	Men	Total
Toronto	2	5	7
Southern Ontario	4	23	27
Quebec	0	2	2
Manitoba	2	1	3
Saskatchewan	–	1	1
British Columbia	1	–	1
Nova Scotia	4	–	4
New Brunswick	0	0	0
Prince Edward Island	0	0	0
Newfoundland	–	1	1
China	–	3	3
Japan	–	1	1
Korea	–	1	1
U.S.A.	1	3	4
U.K.	–	2	2
Unknown	–	3	3
Total	14	46	60

later the United Church, doubled, from 2,114,321 to 4,597,542, comprising one third of Canada's total population. In 1891, the rural population was twice that of the urban centres, but the cumulative effects of the First World War and the resulting industrialization of the economy, as well as the agrarian disasters of the depression in the 1930s, allowed the urban population to gain in numbers until it surpassed the rural population in 1931.

Ontario, with the largest increase in urban population, led the nation in educational reform and development, with a rapid increase in the availability of vocational education in the 1920s. Although postsecondary education remained the privilege of a tiny elite (see table 3), the demands of an increasingly urban population resulted in a rapid increase in educational opportunities.

The expansion of Canadian medical schools from eight in 1911 to ten by 1951 kept pace with the growth of the population, providing approximately one doctor per thousand popula-

TABLE 3
Population of Canada, number of physicians, graduates of medical
schools, university graduates, 1881–1941

Year	Total population of Canada[a]	Total Canadian physicians[b]	Total Canadian Medical graduates[b]	Total University graduates[b]
1881	4,324,810	3,507	–	–
1911	7,206,643	7,411	351	–
1921	8,787,949	8,706	406	3,869
1931	10,376,786	10,020	482	5,804
1941	11,506,655	11,873	562	7,324

Sources:
[a] *Historical Statistics*, Series A 2–14, p. 14
[b] Ibid., Series B 108–15, p. 44
[c] Ibid., Series V 207–14. p. 603 (adapted)

tion from 1881 to 1941, with marginal increases over the
sixty-year period. Physicians comprised a small elite, both
within the population as a whole (the average from 1881 to
1941 was 0.1 per cent) and within the already select group of
university graduates.

Education

Predictably, the majority of volunteers graduated from the
University of Toronto, as this was the hub of the Student
Volunteer Movement in Canada, and Ontario's largest university medical school. Thirty-four, or fifty-six per cent, of the
medical missionaries were Toronto graduates (see table 4).
One medical missionary, who was not a University of Toronto graduate, remarked that his colleagues were constantly
saying, 'In Toronto we did this ...,' and eventually they were
identified as an 'inbred group' with a sense of 'superiority.' A
report on the WCUU by a representative of the Rockefeller
Foundation China Medical Board commented that, 'a reading
of the roster of some of the departments sounds like a roll call
of a University of Toronto alumni association.'[37]

TABLE 4
Medical schools attended by medical missionaries

Institution	Men	Women	Total
U. of Toronto	25	6	31
McGill U.	5	0	5
U. of Manitoba	3	3	6
Queen's U.	4	0	4
U. of Western Ontario	2	1	3
U.S.A. institutions	3	0	3
Dalhousie U.	1	4	5
Edinburgh U.	1	0	1
Unknown	2	0	2
Total	46	14	60

The Flexner Report of 1910, a landmark in the development of American medical schools, rated Canadian medical schools as follows: the University of Toronto and McGill were 'excellent'; the University of Manitoba and Queen's were 'above average'; and the University of Western Ontario and Laval University were 'feeble.'[38] McGill, the first medical school in Canada, was the alma mater of Sir William Osler, whose teaching and textbooks had a profound influence on medical education. The University of Toronto Medical School was an amalgamation of Victoria University, Trinity College, Toronto School of Medicine, and Women's Medical College, and continued to be one of the strongest schools in the country. A comparison of geographic origin and school of graduation, however, indicates that the majority of medical missionaries made a choice of school based primarily on proximity to where they lived.

Medical education was not available to women at the University of Toronto until 1906, or at Queen's until 1943. Only a women's medical college affiliated with Queen's University in Kingston, Ontario, and the Women's Medical College trained women physicians. Outside of these two schools, Dalhousie and the University of Manitoba offered the earliest opportunities for women medical students. Of the fourteen women medical missionaries, six were educated at the University of Toronto, four at Dalhousie, three at Manitoba, and one at the University of Western Ontario.

Medical education prior to the founding of McGill University Medical School in 1824 relied on the apprenticeship system, or foreign medical schools, particularly the University of Edinburgh. The graduates of Edinburgh, who later staffed Canadian medical colleges, brought with them the tradition of clinical training, with emphasis on teaching by lectures, and clinical practice in an associated hospital. The medical curriculum allotted a disproportionately large amount of time to the study of anatomy and physiology, according to the tradition of the European schools. Canadian doctors who pursued postgraduate specialization studied in Britain, France, Germany, Austria, and, after the First World War, the United States. Following the discovery of insulin by Banting and Best in 1921, Canadian medical research came into its own, with the subsequent development of postgraduate opportunities.

For most of the missionaries, specialized training was undertaken during their furlough years, usually in Europe or the United States. A number of the West China Union University medical faculty received fellowships from the Rockefeller Foundation for further study at Peking Union Medical College, usually for several months of the furlough period. Although the missionaries were elites among the population as a whole, they were not an elite group in the medical profession. Only fifteen of the twenty-four had postgraduate training or degrees, and that ratio remained fairly constant during the entire period from 1891 to 1952, even after postgraduate opportunities increased. Most of the medical missionaries went to China immediately after they graduated, and few had the time or money to pursue a postgraduate degree. However, a reliable source external to the mission reported favourably on the professional competence of the medical and dental staff of the university. Regarding the physicians, this source indicated that although 'opportunities for specific training [had] been limited, ... special studies while on furlough,' and experience in the field, upgraded the degree of specialization. Referring to the dental faculty, he

was 'greatly impressed with the type of man on its faculty,
the closeness of their co-operation with one another, and
with the command they seem[ed] to have of their special
field.'[39]

Although a minority held postgraduate degrees, the medical
missionaries were notable as a highly educated group; twenty-
two of them had received degrees in arts, theology, teaching,
or other fields in addition to their medical training; seven
were ordained ministers (five of those recruited between 1891
and 1910), and three were lay ministers.[40]

Socioeconomic Background

In spite of their high level of education, the majority of medical missionaries were not from wealthy families. Between
1894 and 1910 their backgrounds were largely rural, comprising farm families, rural tradesmen, and ministers. Many of the
medical recruits had themselves followed careers in farming
or teaching before they entered the medical profession. During
the period 1911 to 1925 there was a gradual shift towards
those from urban areas, but missionaries came primarily from
ministers' families; two of the recruits were born in China of
missionary parents. During this period there were several missionaries who had served as soldiers in the First World War;
some had been teachers or farmers as well. After 1926 there
was again an increase in urban recruits. Most of the missionaries came from professional or urban merchant backgrounds;
four of them were born in Asian missions to missionary parents, and only one had pursued another occupation prior to
entering medical school. This implies that the postwar medical student's family was financially capable of supporting him
or her through medical school, while in previous years the
prospective student had had to work for several years to prepare financially for the expense of a medical education. Thus,
the trend in medical missionaries' social background shifted
from a rural one to a slightly more affluent urban one, reflecting farmer, working-class, and subsequently merchant and
professional middle-class origins.

Motivations

In his landmark study of American images of Asia, Harold Isaacs reported: 'there must be relatively few people of mature age in this country today [1958] who, if they belong to one of the great Protestant denominations and have been brought up in churchgoing families, have not in some way been touched by the missionary experience. Close kin or family connections, or friends, fellow townsfolk, or fellow students went to China as missionaries. Visiting missionaries back from China appeared quite frequently to tell about their work, ministers and Sunday school teachers spurred their flocks week after week to help in the cause ... Here is where young minds were often scratched most meaningfully and most permanently.'[41] Of the Canadian medical missionaries' responses to the question of motivation to volunteer as a missionary, the most common was the influence of a returned missionary (see table 5).[42] In answer to the question 'What influence led you to offer yourself as a missionary?' one medical missionary replied that returned missionaries had left him with 'a childhood impression growing into a settled conviction.'[43] Another answered: 'Hearing accounts by returned missionaries ... this decision was made when I was about 12 years old and has been confirmed by later contacts with missionaries ...'[44] Thus, the missionary on furlough, travelling across the country with stories and 'lantern shows' to illustrate the plight of poor nations, created deep and lasting impressions in the minds of young Sunday school students.

Although the Student Volunteer Movement, later the Student Christian Movement, was not as potent a force in motivating recruits as contact with returned missionaries, it was still an important factor in the recruitment of medical students to the mission field. Perhaps its appeal rekindled childhood enthusiasms for 'saving the heathen.' In addition, the influence of peer group involvement, and the appealing opportunity for activism, drew the support of young men and women who were at a stage in life when idealism and the desire to better the world were strong motivating forces. An illustra-

TABLE 5
Influences motivating medical missionaries, 1891–1947*

Influenced by	1891–1925	1926–47	Total frequency
Returned missionary	14	11	25
Religion	12	4	16
SVM or SCM	5	7	12
Medical service	6	2	8
Parents	2	4	6
Challenge of China	6	0	6
Total	45	28	73

*Number of respondents 44; see note 42. Figures are based on frequency with which each of the above factors was cited.

tion of this idealism is the response by a medical missionary, who later remarked, that 'Evangelical work was not my job,'[45] in answer to the question of what motivated him to volunteer: 'Desire for greater scope in which to use my abilities than that offered to most medical men in a private practice ... and the desire to be rid of financial worries and aspects that are common to many medical men and other very frequently highly paid professionals.'[46] The influence of the SCM and SVM on this group of medical missionaries increased after 1926 and contributed to the recruitment of half the volunteers between 1926 and 1947.

In the total picture of missionary motivation, religious experience figured second in frequency. As might be expected, the mention of religious motivation dominated the early applications, and it declined somewhat as Canadian society, and the United Church in particular, became more secularized. The early missionary recruits were accepted on the basis that they had undergone the conversion experience, and they had to swear to the fact that they had been 'called by the Holy Spirit to go as a missionary to the heathen.'[47] Later missionaries arrived at their religious convictions of 'the Fatherhood of God' less dramatically, through thought and meditation.[48] Here the medical missionaries differed most significantly from their evangelical counterparts. Implicit, if not stated outright, in their discussions of their 'personal experience in the Christian life'[49] was the controversial belief that the example of the Christian life was as important as, and perhaps more effective than, the actual conversion of non-believers. This belief was expressed in the prevalence of two attitudes among the medical missionaries: 'that the purpose of the missionary enterprise is to bring a more abundant life to as many people as possible,'[50] and that 'the Bible is the most important book for *those of us* who are seeking to know God through Jesus Christ *whose example and teachings are our guide.*'[51] The first statement, from a medical missionary recruit in 1941, reflects the underlying belief, which became more and more prevalent among mission workers, that an influence wider than the salvation of souls was the gift of the medical missions. One missionary stated: 'I felt that my goal was primarily to practice the best scientific medicine that I could practice. Secondarily, if the Chinese felt that something in my religious philosophy was relevant, that was a secondary consideration.'[52]

Even a deeply evangelical medical missionary, who was far more oriented to religion than his contemporaries in the 1940s, expressed the belief that the 'Spirit of Christ and His "Way of Life" could serve as a 'panacea for national as well as personal ills' if they were 'adapted and molded into our international affairs.'[53] Linked to this attitude was the notion that the example of the Christian way of life was as powerful an influence as the actual conversion of individuals. It acknowledged that Christians sought to know God through Christ, implying that other religious beliefs were as legitimate as their own. It was the emphasis on Christian principles, applied to interpersonal relationships, institutions, and national and international politics, that characterized the low-keyed evangelism of the medical missionaries. Almost as a rejection of the notorious conversion of 'rice Christians,' those who came only for the 'loaves and fishes' of the West, one medical missionary stated that for him, preaching to or praying with a patient before surgery was like 'kicking a man when he was down.'[54] It was this belief that one could spread the Christian message by example as well as by teaching that gave the

medical missionaries their raison d'être, which was never
taken for granted, even in the late 1940s, when the medical
work was firmly institutionalized.

Of the other motivating factors mentioned by missionary
applicants, only one stated 'professional interests,' and he was
avowedly secular in his intent and was recruited to serve the
professional needs of the university at a particular time. However, eight of the missionaries signified that providing medical
service was a motivating factor. In most cases, it was only one
of several factors, but the following declarations indicate the
importance of bringing scientific medicine to the Chinese in
the determination of missionary goals. Two of the missionaries studied medicine 'with the intention of becoming a missionary';[55] one saw the role of the missionaries as being 'partners (with the Chinese) in the great enterprise of bringing
healing to the people';[56] another was dedicated to 'winning the
Chinese to an appreciation of good health and care of the
sick.'[57] The identification of science with Christianity is clear
in this statement by the dean of the WCUU College of Dentistry: 'The old beliefs are passing and pass they must as the
Western world brings wider outlooks and scientific logical
reasoning and Christianity to the land.'[58] Only six of the forty-
four mentioned parental influence, and five of these were born
in Asia of missionary parents. The 'challenge of China' was
listed by one-fifth of the applicants before 1910, but even
though the notion of 'our share in Szechuan' persisted, this
appeal disappeared as a conscious motivating factor by 1926.
The word conscious should be stressed here, because the
challenge to Christianize China was incorporated into the
world-view of the United Church of Canada's mission; it was
no longer a novel appeal after 1910, but rather was taken for
granted.

Letters from two of the medical missionaries, recording
their first impressions, provide a valuable insight into their
motivations once they arrived in the field. They are quoted at
length because they vividly portray the sense of challenge
experienced by the missionaries as they left the familiar in
Canada and entered a strange new life. Departing in Novem-

ber of 1933, one missionary wrote: 'Canada's coast gradually
faded and I felt that I had burnt my bridges behind me and it
was up to me to do my best in my new home in China. I
wondered what contribution I would be able to make to her
in the years to come.' After arriving in Chongqing, he wrote:
'The dirt in the streets is amazing ... human and animal
excreta being present wherever you go. The public latrines
also make themselves violently evident to the olfactory sense.
The rats come out in great numbers at night.' In spite of this
dismal picture, this missionary was optimistic about the
future; after attending the Annual Council of Missionaries
meeting in Chengdu, he reported: 'Some of the reports at first
were rather pessimistic and made me feel rather depressed but
later ones were more cheerful and I enjoyed them better. The
work seemed to be in a pretty healthy condition on the whole
and I was quite thrilled to be able to count myself one of the
body that was meeting there.'[59] This enthusiasm was evident
in the letter of another medical missionary who felt the same
challenge to contribute to change in China: 'As one walks the
streets of the various cities and towns one is very much
impressed with the need for sanitary measures ... then too the
need for surgical treatment of those suffering from tumours,
deformities and curable eye disorders is everywhere apparent.
There is certainly no dearth of work for the medical man ...
It is a wonderful adventure, this bringing of Christianity to
the Chinese not alone as a religion, but in its relation to living and the spiritual force which will change their lives.'[60]

Professional Ideology

Having examined the medical missionaries' social background
and motivations, one must also consider their professional
ideology, the legacy of the historical development of their
profession. The following analysis provides a perspective on
the development of the ideals and attitudes of the medical
missionaries as doctors.

In the Middle Ages, 'medical missionary' might have
seemed a contradiction in terms. Theology was considered a

higher branch of knowledge than natural science. The philo-
sopher-priest ministered to the soul, while the physician ministered to the body.[61] The earliest hospitals were, in fact,
religious institutions created to care for the poor and sick.
Although secular involvement increased from the thirteenth
century, when Western European municipal authorities took
over responsibility for the care of the indigent population,
hospitals remained custodial centres, with no concern for
curative work and no need for the medical profession. It was
not until the Industrial Revolution of the mid-nineteenth
century that the relationship between disease and the social
life of the community was recognized. As 'public-spirited'
citizens developed social conscience, they urged local authorities to accept responsibility for improving public welfare.[62]
The concept of public health and civic sanitation developed
as a consequence of this recognition, and national legislation
to provide health care was first introduced in 1881 in Germany by Bismarck. This example was soon followed on a
smaller scale by Britain, Canada, and the United States, where
municipal governments became involved in the public health
movement.[63] It was during this time that doctors began to
emerge as civic leaders.[64] In Ontario in 1882, the first Provincial Board of Health appointed physicians as provincial health
officers with powers to enforce quarantine, epidemic controls,
and public sanitation.[65]

The late nineteenth-century discoveries of the germ theory
of disease by Pasteur and Koch gave medicine a scientific
thrust, and, combined with the practical achievements of
technological developments, surgery, and asepsis, gave rise to
modern medicine.[66] No longer an itinerant herbalist with
nebulous principles for diagnosis and treatment, the doctor
became part of an increasingly sophisticated profession, with
its technological skills, professional schools, code of dress, and
aura of authority. At the same time, however, herbalists and
unqualified practitioners continued to care for the health
needs of the poorer classes, who could not afford the luxury
of academic scientific medicine.[67]

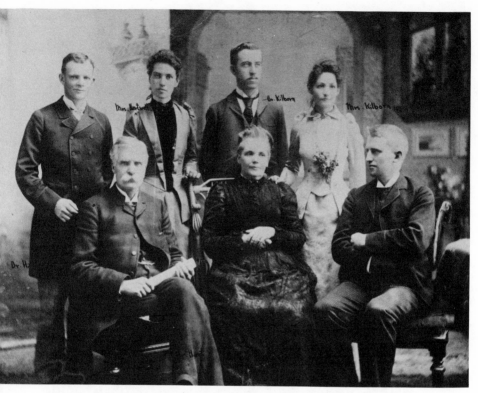

The first group of Methodist missionaries in Sichuan, 1891,
included Drs Omar and Retta Gifford Kilborn.

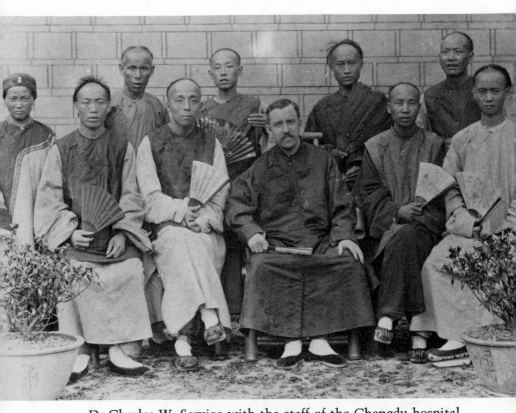

Dr Charles W. Service with the staff of the Chengdu hospital,
c. 1897

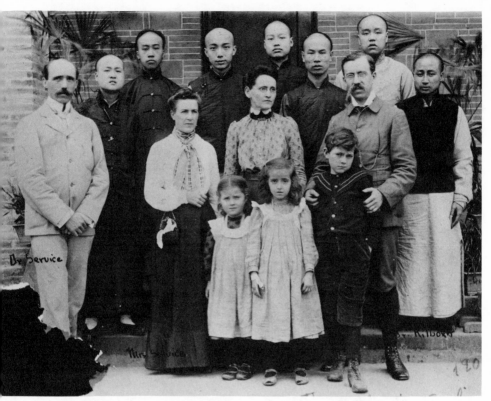

The first Canadian medical missionaries in Sichuan: Dr and Mrs
C.W. Service, Drs Omar and Retta Gifford Kilborn and their
children, Cora, Constance, and Leslie, 1904

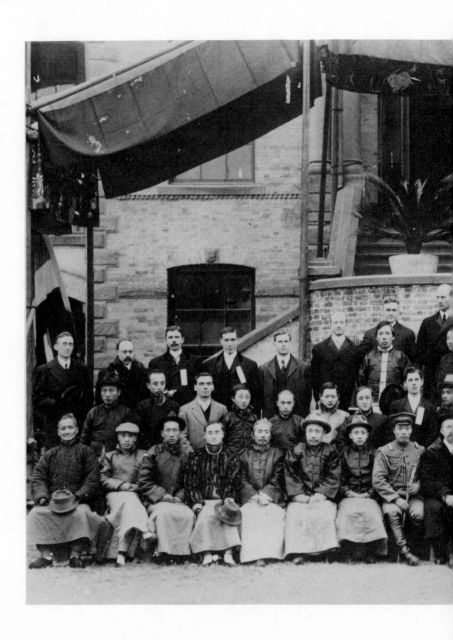

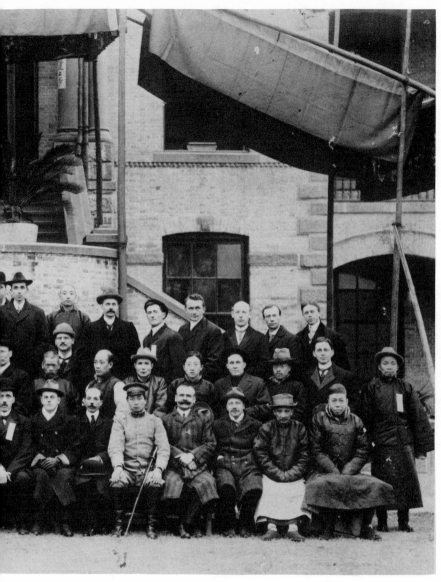

Opening of the Si Sheng Ci Men's Hospital, Chengdu, 30 January 1913. It was attended by representatives of the foreign diplomatic community, the government of Sichuan, local gentry, and missionaries. Dr O.L. Kilborn is in the front row centre.

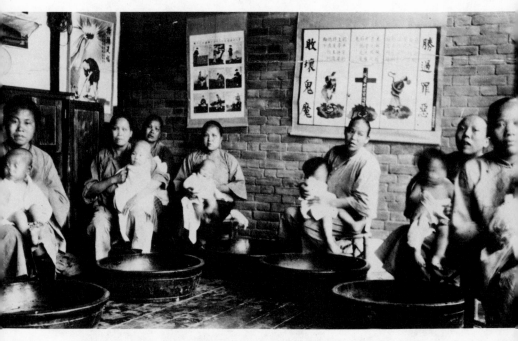

A baby welfare clinic at the Fuzhou mission station. This was an important aspect of mission hospital work outside the university, from the early 1900s to 1949.

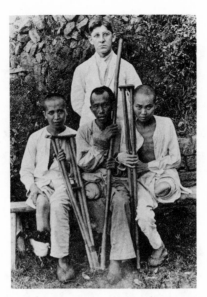

Dr Frank F. Allan with patients, at Renshow, one of the ten West China Mission stations, 1917

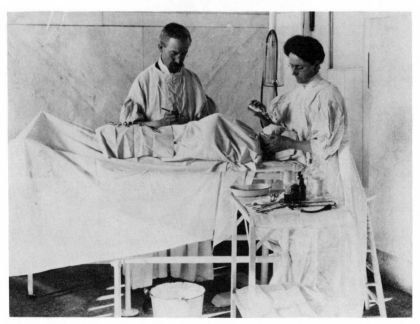

Drs Omar and Retta Gifford Kilborn in the operating room of the Rongxian station hospital, c. 1918

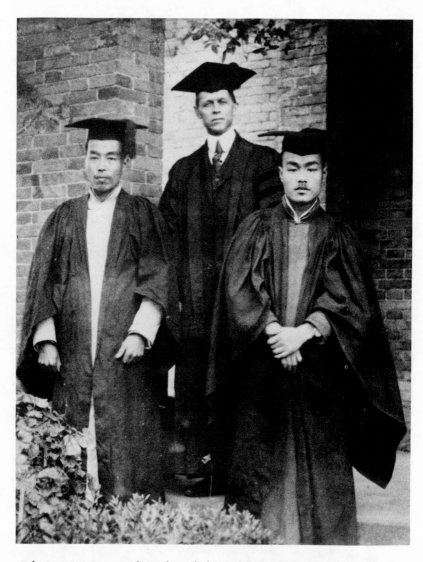

Edwin N. Meuser, founder of the School of Pharmacy, with the
first graduates of the school, early 1920s

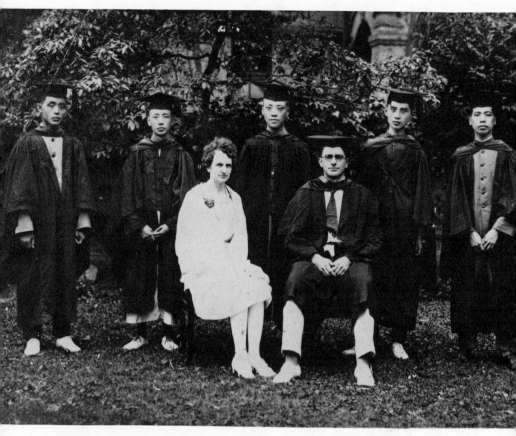

One of the first graduating classes in medicine, 1926. From left to right: L.H. Chen, D.D. Yuan, T.D. Fay, S.D. Du, G.B. Loh, Dr and Mrs Best (The first class had only one graduate, Dr Liu, who entered in 1914 and graduated in 1921.)

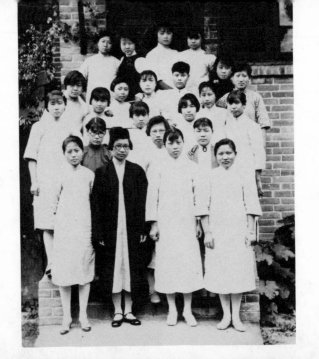

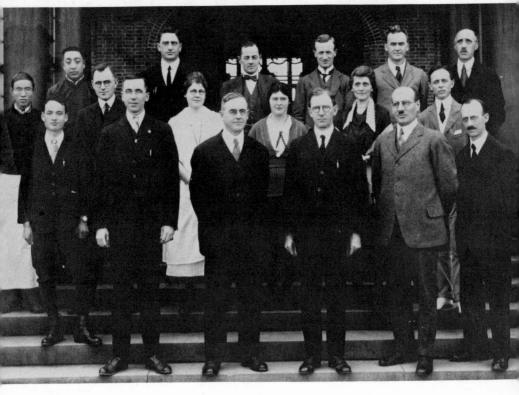

This picture, taken in 1934, includes the five women members of the class of 1937 (total, thirteen students) and the first woman graduate, Dr Helen Yoh, class of 1932.

The medical faculty of the WCUU, 1923. From left to right, front row: Drs Hsiao, Wilford, Morse (Dean), Beech (President), Kelly, Thompson; middle row: Mr Chang, Drs L. and J. Kilborn, Miss Downer, Dr R. Kilborn, E.N. Meuser; back row: Drs Chien, Best, Humphreys, Stubbs, Mr Bayne, Dr C.W. Service

Dr Lincoln Dsang (Zhang Lin-gao) and family, 1932. He was the first Chinese president of WCUU. His eldest daughter is a professor at the medical university of Chengdu.

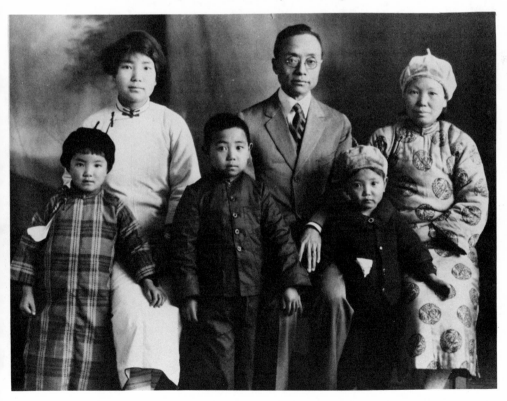

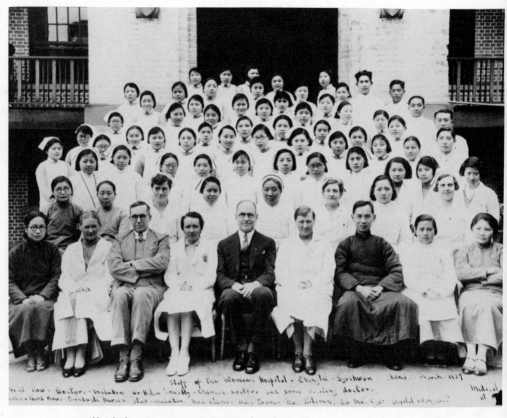

Staff of the Women's Hospital, Chengdu, 1937. Many of the nurses and doctors were graduates of WCUU, including Drs Helen Yoh and Ruth Zhang.

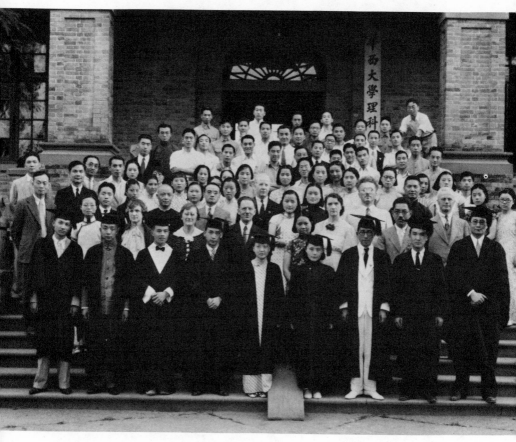

Dentistry professors, graduates, and students, 1938 (Dr H. Mullett, third row centre). The photo inscription attests to the capability and suitability of Chinese young women as dentists: they are 'much gentler than "some" of the men dentists ... are not taking second place ... not afraid of hard work ... a tremendous blessing to their own countrywomen.'

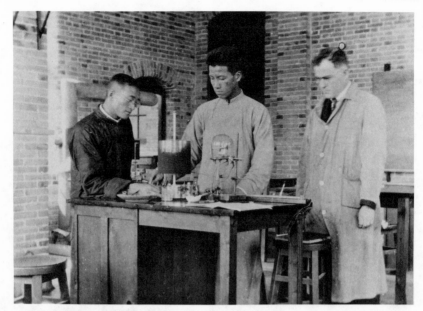

Dr Leslie Kilborn, Professor of Physiology and later Dean of Medicine, in laboratory with students, c. 1930

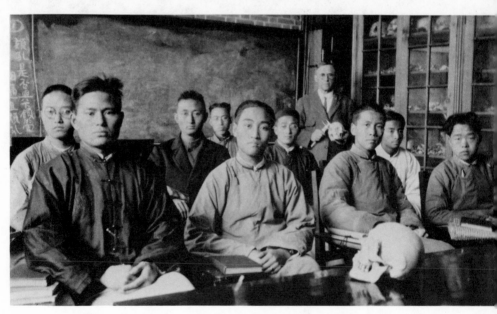

Dr W.R. Morse's anatomy class; this group graduated in 1931.

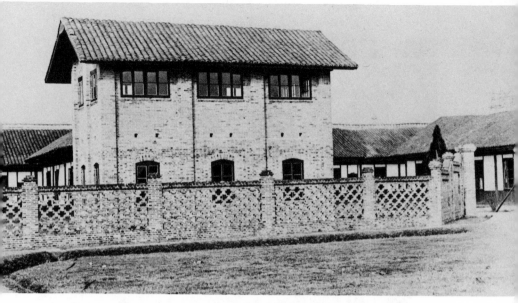

The first building used as a medical college, West China Union University, Chengdu, c. 1919. A new and much larger building was constructed in the mid-1920s.

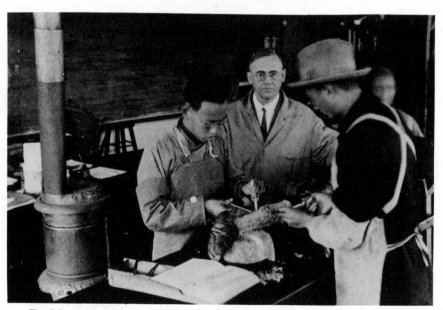

Dr Morse instructing students in dissection, early 1920s, in the first medical college building

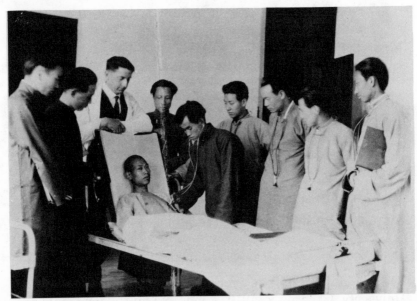

Dr C. Best instructing students on the use of the
stethoscope, 1930s

Dr J.E. Thompson, one of the first professors of dentistry, with
student and patient, c. 1920s

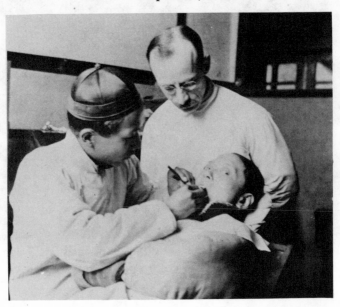

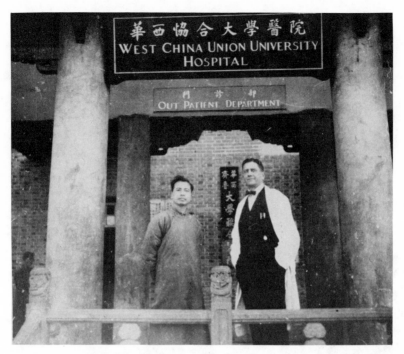

Dr Luo Guang-bi and Dr Best in front of the university hospital, late 1930s. Dr Luo's daughter is at present Vice-Dean of Dentistry at WCUMS in Chengdu.

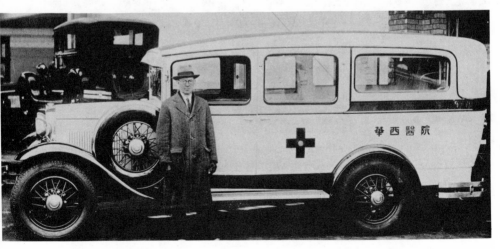

In the late 1940s, Dr Joseph Beech returned to the university with funds and other relief, including the donation of an ambulance.

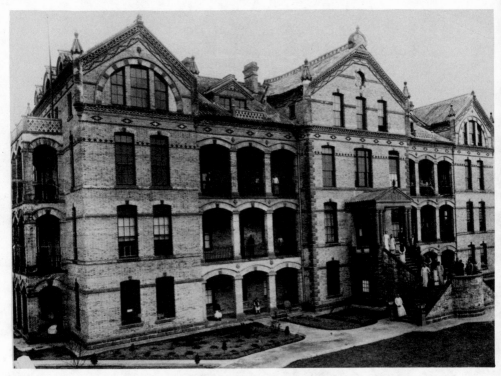

The Si Sheng Ci Men's Hospital, built by the Methodists, c. 1913 (see the earlier picture also). After 1949 it served as the Second Municipal People's Hospital, until the early 1970s; in 1993 it was demolished and replaced by a surgical hospital.

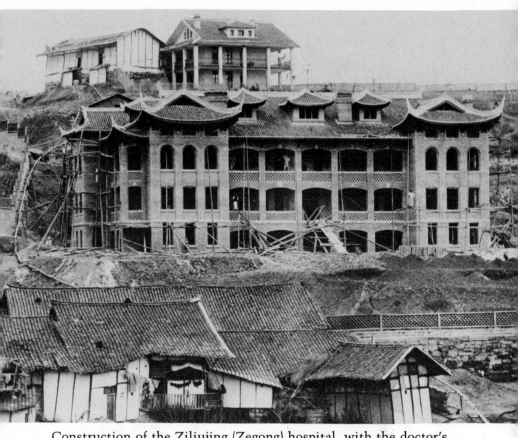

Construction of the Ziliujing (Zegong) hospital, with the doctor's
residence on the hill behind, 1916

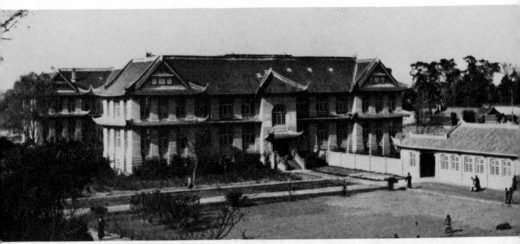

Teaching hospital, WCUU Medical-Dental College, c. 1942

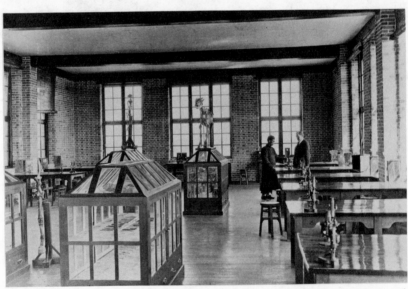

Dr Morse with a student in the WCUU biology building, now used
as the anatomy building, c. 1930

The president's residence, built in 1924, currently serves as one of the WCUMS guest-houses.

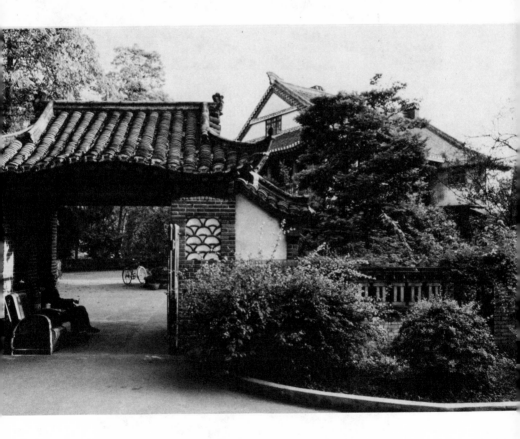

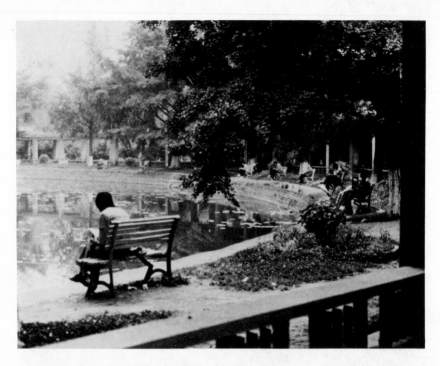

In spite of its tumultuous history, the campus still stands as an island of tranquillity in bustling Chengdu. The lotus pond, designed in the 1920s to provide a meditative sanctuary for students, is still much appreciated by students, staff, and families who live on the WCUMS campus.

Dr Helen Yoh (Yue Yichen), the first woman to graduate from WCUU, in 1932. She is still consulted by the Obstetrics and Gynaecology Department at the medical school in Chengdu.

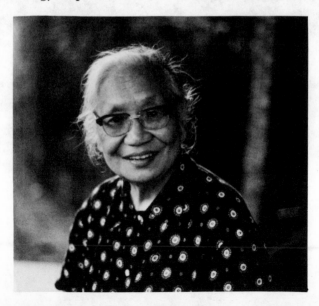

Canadian patients in the late nineteenth century were served both by itinerant 'doctors,' and by physicians trained in European and, later, Canadian medical schools. There was no government regulation of medical practice or training. It was not until 1922 that the federal government passed the Canada Medical Act, appointing the Medical Council of Canada to issue the licentiate examination.[68] The Canadian Medical Association (CMA), organized in the early 1920s by graduate physicians, initially sought to enforce uniform standards of medical education and to control the proliferation of unqualified practitioners. On the one hand, this professional association exerted pressure on government to legislate public-health measures; on the other, its members reacted to the introduction of health insurance schemes in continental Europe and Great Britain with varying degrees of hostility. The CMA disapproved of government control of their profession, but at the same time encouraged government responsibility for the nation's health.

Perhaps the outstanding characteristic of medical practice in Canada, prior to the intense urbanization and centralization of medical care which followed the Second World War, was the self-reliance forced upon medical practitioners isolated by Canadian geography and climate. The scarcity of educated men and women in a predominantly rural nation led to the elevated status of the physicians as the learned members of the rural community. They often served as 'minister, merchant, physician, as well as farmer and mechanic.' At the same time, a rural physician's description of his practice reveals the limitations of patients' knowledge about health and the limited expectations the public had of scientific medicine: 'I found a people thinking in, trusting in, and acting on superstitions of long ago, and fatalistic, who held it as a token of ignorance that one was unwilling to diagnose and prescribe without first examining the patient, and still more so that one might advise observation before labelling an uncertain case; who had no temper for continuous treatment, whose ultimate therapy was the bottle of 'doctor's medicine'; and who, if this

from the hands of four or five doctors of neighbourhood re-
pute, failed, regarded themselves as incurable; all advice as to
conduct of living held valueless.'[69] This situation, of geographic isolation and a superstitious populace, was not unlike the
situation which the missionaries encountered in Sichuan
Province. While their urban-based education did not prepare
them for the harsh realities of medical practice in China, the
tradition of the independent self-reliance of the general practitioner was some preparation.

The development of the dental profession exhibited the
same trends as that of medicine. Dentistry became profession-
alized as technology and science contributed to its effectiveness, and dental education first became associated with a
university in 1906.[70] Like medicine, dentistry was a self-regu-
lating profession with a national coordinating body, the
Canadian Dental Association, established in 1902. Although
Canadian dentists espoused the values of public health and
preventive dentistry, and Ontario appointed a Director of
Dental Services to the Provincial Board of Health in 1924,
the profession remained strongly individualistic. Professional
services remained on a private enterprise basis, and government regulation was consistently rejected.

The dilemma inherent in the ideology of both the medical
and the dental professions has been the association of doctors
and dentists with the hospital, a public, community institution, and public health, a function of government, in opposition to their closely guarded professional autonomy.[71] A study
of the medical professional roles suggests that Western doctors
view themselves as exemplars of moral standards and social
conscience, while at the same time maintaining their independence from the 'State behemoth'. Physicians have been
successful in maintaining their independence through para-
governmental agencies (the Colleges of Medicine and Dentistry and the Canadian Medical and Dental Associations).
The source of professional rejection of state control at the
same time as the profession seeks government support is
attributed to the following paradox: 'The patronage and state
mediation of science helps to explain a seeming paradox that

the growth of scientific expertise, while increasing the prestige and legitimacy of science itself, has been associated with a decline in the power and prestige of individual scientists.[72]

In sum, we can see the emergence in the West of a paternalistic profession, striving to maintain high standards of scientific research and technology along with professional autonomy, and at the same time lobbying for an expanded government role in the field of health care.

Summary and Conclusion

As the concept of the ideal medical missionary evolved from evangelist doctor to medical educator, the missionary recruits reflected an increasing degree of professionalization and specialization. From 1910 to 1940, the requirements for 'missionary zeal' became less stringent, while those for professional and social competence became more important.

In terms of their social background, the medical missionaries represented an Ontario-born and -educated elite, although they were not an economic elite. As doctors, they were committed to science, with its rational, logical methods and technology, and to humanitarianism, the basis of their professional creed. They reflected the paternalism of their profession, which had the authority vested in knowledge and the historical precedent of the role of moral exemplar. Their resistance to government intervention in the practice of their profession, in spite of their professional influence on the expansion of government responsibility for public health, defines them as conservatives who supported the status quo. This was the paradox in medical missionary perceptions: they sought to change the Chinese social and political system, but were inherently resistant to change in their own profession.

The motivating forces that led the individual medical missionaries to volunteer for the West China Mission reflected the influence of the SVM. This movement not only enlisted the college youth of North America in the support of the missions, but made a particular appeal to the needs in China. The mission strategy from the late 1880s, when the move-

ment was founded, to the outbreak of the First World War,
emphasized the Christianization of an indigenous elite who
would in turn evangelize their fellow countrymen. After 1914
the strategy shifted to an emphasis on establishing Christian
leaders in the community and nation, with evangelization to
follow national development gradually.[73] As Christians, the
medical missionaries held the fundamental belief that personal transformation was the path to personal salvation, but
as members of the United Church, they emphasized social
responsibility as the goal of Christian enterprise.

The policy that derived from these influences was the concentration of medical efforts in the development of the Chinese medical profession. 'The multiplication of ourselves' was
the watchword of the medical missionaries, who thus sought
to maximize their influence in the transformation of China
into a modern nation. As agents of change, they envisioned
themselves as Christian men and women of science, imbued
with the values of Christ-like humanitarianism and scientific
rationality, and the principles of Western democratic liberal-
ism.

John King Fairbank's description of the American Protestant
missionaries of this century could apply equally to their Canadian counterparts. He portrayed them as possessing 'personal
responsibility for one's own character and conduct; an optimistic belief in progress toward general betterment, especially
through the use of education, invention and technology; and
a conviction of moral and cultural worth, at times even superiority, justified both by the religious teachings of the Holy
Bible and by the political principles of the Founding Fathers.'[74]

The profile of Canadian medical missionaries that emerges
is one of individuals who were devoted to Christian principles, but reluctant to preach the Gospel as a means of evangelizing the non-Christian world. Influenced by their scientific
medical training, the missionaries were convinced of the
superiority of a rational application of science and technology.
The fellowship of the Christian student associations tempered
the missionaries' religious beliefs by the emphasis on social
action and on the moral principles of brotherhood, humanitar-

ianism, and selfless dedication. As Canadians and as Christians, they believed in the Western political ethic of equality of opportunity and the rights of individuals to the benefits of modern science and technology. This identification of the benefits of Western civilization with the 'Kingdom of God' was fundamental to the missionaries' perception of their goals. These men and women were scientific missionaries, and their powerful vision was the revitalization of China.

The 'Receivers': Chinese Students at the College of Medicine and Dentistry

Alumni: Sources of Information

The medical missionaries delivered Western medical education to a cohort of Chinese students who were moulded by a range of social, political, and cultural influences. This chapter assesses the Chinese students of the WCUU College of Medicine and Dentistry in terms of the social and political context in which they lived: their individual socioeconomic backgrounds, their careers as students, their professional careers after graduation and before the establishment of the People's Republic of China.

Between 1920 and 1949, 579 men and women graduated from the West China Union University College of Medicine and Dentistry. At the time of this study, most of the 1920s generation of alumni are deceased; the alumni from provinces outside of Sichuan are scattered throughout China. The majority of those who graduated in the 1940s either stayed abroad after completing their postgraduate studies or fled the Communist regime after 1949 for societies that were more hospitable to educated elites. It is estimated that fifty to sixty-five per cent of graduates left China between 1949 and 1950.[1] Based on the more conservative estimate of a fifty per cent emigration rate, and taking into account that there were forty graduates in the 1920s who may no longer be alive, it is postulated that there are approximately 250 to 300 alumni still in China; undoubtedly, some of them are no longer alive.

The challenge of locating these alumni was to find appropriate individuals who had access to their names and to gain introduction through a third party. This was achieved in 1986, and by 1988 the president of the newly formed Alumni Association of the West China University of Medical Sciences (renamed from Sichuan Medical College in 1985, to celebrate the school's seventy-fifth anniversary) provided a list of 128 names and addresses of alumni in China.[2] A questionnaire (see the appendix for the English version) was mailed from within China to the eighty-eight alumni outside the West China campus. Those on campus were interviewed, and the questionnaire was filled in by either the author or the respondent. The total return rate of the questionnaires was fifty-one, or forty per cent. This sample represents eighteen per cent of the estimated alumni population in China. A total of thirty-one interviews augmented the questionnaire data.

Other information about the alumni was obtained from an additional eighteen interviews, six with alumni now in the United States, and twelve with individuals in China who were or are affiliated with the university. This figure includes interviews with several university administrators and alumni of other faculties. In November 1989 three interviews were conducted with alumni in Hong Kong, and the author met with a group of four alumni in Shanghai. A total of forty-four alumni were interviewed.

The questionnaire sought to gather data about socioeconomic background, student life, career after graduation, and attitudes to medical modernization. Many of the questions had an unavoidable similarity to the questions typical of political interrogation in the People's Republic of China, which integrates private and public life into a politically sensitive whole. The author was surprised at the candour of many of the respondents, particularly in the interviews. Considering the caution exercised by traditional Chinese in communicating with a stranger and a foreigner, this method of data collection, although fraught with complications, proved to be very rewarding.

Interview data were corroborated with archival material
collected at both the United Church of Canada Archives in
Toronto and the West China University of Medical Sciences
Archives in Chengdu. It is not possible to make systematic
use of the Chengdu archives; however, considerable information on student backgrounds and university relations was
available. The archival, interview, and survey data represent
the 1930s and 1940s generations of alumni.[3] There is relatively little information on the 1920s generation.

Socioeconomic Background of Students

It should have been evident from the list of alumni received
that two categories defined the subgroups within this cohort.
The list was arranged by geographic location; within each
geographic location, it was arranged by year of graduation. A
meeting in Chengdu, with a senior physician who offered to
assist in arranging the interview schedule, reinforced the
notion that year of graduation was an important factor in
classifying the alumni. The interviews were arranged by 'generation,' beginning with the 1930s generation, and proceeding
to the 1940s generation, ending with the youngest of the
alumni groups on campus. It also became clear from the interviews that there were two basic geographic categories: Sichuanese alumni, and 'downriver' alumni.

Although the early data were not available, it is assumed
that the majority of students in the 1920s and early 1930s were
from Sichuan. Chengdu was too remote to attract students
from other parts of China. By 1937, however, with the Japanese occupation of North and East China, increasing numbers
of students took refuge in Sichuan. In 1937, thirty-four per
cent of medical students were from outside Sichuan.[4] By 1946,
refugee students had swelled the non-Sichuanese population
to sixty-three per cent.[5] By 1947, most had returned to their
homes in other parts of China. Although students reported
that they chose their associates based on their faculty of study,
there is anecdotal evidence that the social and dialect differences between Sichuanese students and those from 'downriver'

created some social distance between the groups. Furthermore, the Cantonese students were considered a special group because of the differences in dialect and food preferences. In terms of the long-term integration of the groups, very few 'downriver' students remained in Sichuan after the war. It is a tradition in China to return to one's place of birth.

The first students to enter the medical college in the 1920s came from poor families, and they were subsidized by the missionaries.[6] In fact, missionary building plans for the college dormitories took into consideration the notion that campus living standards should not be higher than what the students would be able to afford after graduation. In time, many more students from affluent families enrolled in the college, as it became evident to middle-class families that medicine and dentistry were desirable careers.

The survey data suggest that half of the alumni came from intellectual families (twenty-three of forty-six). This correlates with student records in the campus archives indicating that forty-eight per cent of students came from families where the fathers were doctors, teachers, engineers, clergy, lawyers, or officials.[7] The difference between the 1937–8 group of refugee students and the other survey respondents, who were predominantly 1940s graduates, is the larger number of merchant families in the former group (twenty per cent compared with seven per cent). This could be explained by the fact that the former group was largely Sichuanese, while the latter included many children of intellectual families in the coastal cities. Only a small percentage of students were from military families (three per cent and seven per cent, respectively), and from peasant families (thirteen per cent and four per cent, respectively).

The families of the alumni were remarkable for their dedication to higher education. Of the alumni surveyed, eighty per cent had siblings who went to university; ninety per cent of the siblings were employed in 'intellectual' occupations. Considering that they reported the data for up to eight siblings, this is a high rate. Spouses of alumni were likely chosen from among classmates, as fifty-five per cent of the spouses were

also physicians or dentists, and forty-seven per cent attended
the same university. Data on education and occupation of the
children of alumni indicate that the same appreciation for
higher education and intellectual occupations continued to
the next generation, as ninety-two to ninety-seven per cent
attended university, and eighty-nine per cent were employed
as intellectuals (about one-third of these in medicine).[8]

Both the survey data and the archival data indicate that the
majority of alumni attended government or missionary primary schools, with an increase in enrolment at missionary
schools beginning at the junior high school level. The availability of English-language instruction at missionary schools,
and the mission policy of recruiting university entrants from
their own middle schools, likely influenced this trend.[9]

Religious Background of Students

The religious profile of students shows some consistency in
generational affiliation with Christianity. In the survey
results, fifty-one per cent reported Christian grandparents,
and fifty-three per cent reported Christian parents. Only
twenty-eight of the fifty-one respondents answered the question concerning religious affiliation. Ten of these identified
themselves as Christians, while eighteen indicated no affiliation. The lack of response on the part of the others can be
interpreted as either an unwillingness to record religious
affiliation on paper or an indication that there was no religious affiliation. In any case, a minority of alumni reporting
in the 1988 survey identified themselves as Christians.
Earlier data from the university archives record thirty-five
per cent of the medical students in 1946 as Christian, compared with sixteen per cent of the total university student
population at WCUU;[10] another source reports thirty-eight per
cent, or 87 of 230.[11] Given the circumstances of religious
persecution, it is understandable that so few alumni in the
People's Republic of China have maintained religious affilia-
tions that they would be willing to record on a survey questionnaire.

Student Life: Culture, Social Life, and Politics

Most of the students at WCUU reported limited involvement
in extracurricular activities because of the demands of medical study.[12] However, during the 1940s, many joined the university choir, and ballroom dancing was popular. The Hong
Kong refugees were credited with introducing the sound of the
'big bands' of the 1940s. Only the waltz and the foxtrot were
approved of by the missionaries – the jitterbug and the tango
were considered too risqué. Another source of entertainment
was supplied by the American GI's stationed close to the
campus. They passed on cheap novels to the students, with
detective stories being especially popular[13].

The missionaries held open-house receptions on a rotating
basis, each one hosting about fifteen students for tea, biscuits,
and classical music. The appeal may have been the biscuits,
as many students during the 1940s had limited food budgets.
During the 1930s, and into the 1940s, these missionary receptions were associated with Bible study as well.

Two sources in the archives provide descriptive information
about the students' social values. One source was a set of
profiles composed by the class of 1943, each writing a short
passage about a fellow student. These are replete with references to trustworthy friends, exceptional academic talent,
social commitment, and patriotic zeal. Many of the passages
are written in classical style, with numerous literary and
historical allusions, demonstrating that this generation of
Chinese students had the benefit of both a traditional Chinese
and a modern Western education. In one profile, a classmate
teases his friend for having a domineering girlfriend. He refers
to him as 'third elder brother ... historically Su Tung-po
feared his wife; he was the third in his family.'[14]

A second, detailed description of personal values appears in
the 1944 student applications, where students had to answer
questions about themselves pertaining to the following categories: their families, childhood, school life, interests, motivation, political ideas, personality, aspirations, attitude
towards school life, attitudes towards marriage and the oppo-

site sex, social activities, people they loved and hated, study plans, and determination to overcome difficulties. Most of these[15] mentioned the student's abhorrence of hypocrisy, greed, and 'slimy characters.' The words *frankness* and *honesty* appeared repeatedly in their applications. Many admired the May Fourth generation of Chinese professors who had attained a high level of Western education. Most reported that they were motivated by a desire to serve the sick, to be respected professionally, to be useful, and to have an autonomous profession. This accords with the survey data.

There were only three women in the class of 1943. One was nicknamed 'Clever Orchid'; another, who was referred to as the most popular girl in the class, had as her motto, 'Today's Business Is Today's Work.' The third was praised for having not only superior clinical skills, but also the potential to be 'a very talented and creative housewife,' which anyone would know who had tasted her homemade pig's head![16]

The first woman student, Yue Yichen (Helen Yoh), was admitted into the university in 1932. A member of the second generation of West China medical students, she came from a conservative Sichuanese family. Her story is illustrative. She was born into a family typical of early twentieth century China – an extended family living in a four-sided courtyard home. Yichen had ten brothers and sisters, and with all the cousins in her extended family, the courtyard was home to sixteen children. As a young child, she felt frustrated watching her mother care for sick family members. She was determined to learn the skills that would allow her to alleviate the suffering and death which she witnessed in the family home.

Yichen's father was an affluent merchant. Like other Sichuanese families of the time, he encouraged his children to acquire the skills that would allow them to survive and prosper in a rapidly changing social environment. The traditional route to success had been dismantled with the abolition of the civil service examinations in 1905. The end of the Qing dynasty in 1911 terminated the bureaucratic system of meritocracy. Emerging power holders had different skills. For this new generation, it was military prowess that allowed them to challenge the contenders for political and economic control. But economic strength could also be derived from a new source: the knowledge of science and foreign languages. In the coastal cities, the new republic encouraged the development of modern industry and commerce, adopting the ways of the Western imperialist powers as the path to 'wealth and power.' Although missionary schools had been the initial source of modern scientific education, cosmopolitan centres like Shanghai, Peking, Tienstin, and Canton had developed indigenous schools that offered the new, 'modern' curriculum. This went beyond the anachronistic Chinese classics to teach English, French, German, geography, mathematics, science, and physical education. In Sichuan, where missionary institutions developed later and in more isolation than their coastal counterparts, there were fewer opportunities for Western education. The missionary schools were the primary route to Western learning, and hence the skills that promised a secure livelihood in an unknown future. Western medicine in particular offered a profession that was perceived as independent of the vagaries of political conflict. The medical profession, with its provision of an essential service, was more autonomous, and more lucrative, than either the traditional occupations or the modern vocations.

Like other individuals in Sichuan's emergent middle class in the late nineteenth century, Yichen's grandfather embraced Christianity, joining an American Baptist Church. The entire family became Christians, and her uncle was appointed director of one of the dormitories at the WCUU. It was this connection that facilitated Yichen's entrance into the university's middle school, a step which almost guaranteed her admission to the university upon graduation.

Although girls in urban, affluent families at the turn of the century had more opportunities to attend school than their less prosperous counterparts, it was extremely rare for a woman to enter university. Even in the West, where the missionary educators hailed from, women were segregated into the rare medical schools established for women only. It was exceptional to find women medical students who attended medical college with men. Yichen was the first woman to be admitted to the West China College of Medicine in 1932. For the first three years of her training, as the only woman in her class, she was in the constant company of a chaperone, usually one of the missionary wives. Over the next seventeen years, only twenty-six women students attended WCUU medical school. This rate was lower than that of metropolitan schools in North and East China, where, as early as 1924, for example, Qilu University had forty-two women medical students because of its amalgamation with the North China Medical College for Women.[17] Like many of this group, Dr Yue Yichen married a classmate with whom she could share her professional goals and interests.

In spite of her commitment to her profession, Yichen was still motivated by the pragmatic considerations of a traditional wife and mother. She originally chose ophthalmology as her specialty, rejecting the urging of her professors to specialize in obstetrics and gynaecology. She reasoned that the lifestyle of such a profession was not suitable for a woman, although she was entreated to serve the needs of Sichuan's women. This appeal failed to convince her, but when the professor of obstetrics, Gladys Cunningham, offered her the prospect of a fellowship abroad, the young doctor changed her mind and set off to study in Canada, England, and the United States for the next decade, until her return to China in 1950.

As a group, the students at the university were conservative. Although they evacuated the school during the 1925 anti-Christian movement, they did so under threat of attack from militant radicals who accused them of being 'foreign slaves'.[18] The Student Body (the name of the student association) issued a manifesto condemning the Wanxian incident and British imperialism, and the university was closed for a week.[19] At the end of the week the students voted to end the strike, and one relieved faculty member attributed this to the influence of the missionaries, and the stability of the students, which allowed them to resist 'Red' pressure. Following the strike, parents of students placed an announcement 'in some of the

leading papers' of Chengdu, condemning the strike and supporting the university. They argued that the WCUU was
superior to government schools because it was 'not affected by
changes in the government,' and that the foreigners do not
'invade through education,' but rather provide otherwise un-
available opportunities for higher education in West China.[20]
Several members of the medical faculty described the student
outbursts as misdirected frustration, calling the agitators
'ignorant, insolent, pitiful, misinformed, and helpless against
the (Chinese) military.'[21] Another assessment characterized
the students in the movement as an 'undisciplined, ununited
bunch of zealots – they want reform but have not the direct-
ing mind and organizing genius to procure any effective measures – I might add they lack a little conviction backed by a
stiff back bone.'[22]

At the same time, the first group of medical students completed their training, and Dr E.R. Cunningham expressed his
pride in this group of graduates, saying, 'We are full of hopes
that they will do lots for their country and be a credit to the
institution which gave them their training.'[23]

The conservative nature of the students was sometimes
interpreted by their peers in government institutions as lack
of patriotism. In response to this accusation, some of the
WCUU students 'advocated direct military preparation and
training' to combat the Japanese invasion of Manchuria in
1931. They were urged by the faculty to concentrate on their
studies and thus ensure their future contribution to solving
China's problems; the students decided to continue classes
and raise funds for Red Cross war relief to demonstrate their
patriotism.[24] Dr R. Spooner, dormitory principal of Hart College in 1935, reported that the 'national crisis' had given students a 'new sense of national loyalty,' but that personal
problems frequently created tension, as old and new morality
conflicted.[25] Dr Collier stated that the Chinese students were
'materialistic, and see Science only from that viewpoint.'[26] It
was generally agreed that most students were not politically
active but concerned with their studies and the acquisition of
their professional degrees. One student who attended the

university indicated that private university students such as
many of those at WCUU came from well-to-do families who
could afford the fees; the government universities on the
other hand were subsidized. He suggested that students who
joined the Nationalist Party (Guomindang) did so for financial
support and 'to get into the system' so that 'after they graduated they can get a position.' Student unions were mainly
for recreational activities, and most students were apolitical.[27]
A professor in the dental college reported that the politically
active students were members of the fascist *Sanminzhuyi*
Youth Corps, a branch of the Guomindang, and this group
accounted for only a handful of students.[28] Student affiliation
with the Communists was never reported, but this activity
would have been extremely guarded since the Guomindang
was committed to destroying Communist influence. Although
arts students tended to be involved in politics, science students were generally characterized as pragmatic and apolitical.

Political affiliation as reported in the alumni survey data
was very low. Other than the Communist Party, political
parties in China are more form than substance, with no real
political power. Membership in any political party has traditionally been clandestine, with a minority of members broad-
casting their party affiliation. In the survey, only eighteen of
forty-one responded to the question regarding their political
affiliation before 1949, and twenty-two of forty-one answered
the question for post-1949 political membership. Of the pre-
1949 group, two were members of the Guomindang, and the
rest claimed no affiliation. After 1950, four joined the Communist Party, twelve belonged to one of the democratic
parties, and of these, seven (twenty-two per cent) belonged to
the intellectual September Third Party.

The attitude of the 1943 class towards politics, as reported
in their application forms, is congruent with the survey data,
in that the students emphasized patriotic sentiments rather
than ideological commitment. Some gave cursory mention to
the ubiquitous Three People's Principles of Sun Yat-sen: nationalism, democracy, and the people's livelihood. One answer

expressed the apolitical nature of the medical students quite clearly: 'N/A – a science student.'[29]

Political activities on campus were rare until the influx of refugee students after 1938. Even then, communist activities were underground, especially after 1941.[30] Although there were political sympathies for both sides among the faculty, medical students did not indicate that faculty members tried to influence their political beliefs. The only incident which was reported by a number of informants was the influence of one Chinese professor in the faculty of dentistry who was a member of the *Sanminzhuyi* Youth Corps. He reportedly was responsible for the arrest and execution of a woman student accused of being a Communist. There were also several accusations that student discipline was discriminatory, favouring members of the Youth Corps. It is notable that this faculty member had little overt support from his colleagues or students. A report in the *University Bulletin* details his participation in a summer medical service program in the Sichuan countryside. In the organizational chart, he appears as the director of medical services, the keeper of the supplies office, the director of the medical branch hospital, and the head of the dental department. There are no other familiar alumni names on the chart, indicating that although he was the one individual who had political influence, he was fairly isolated within the College.[31]

The present university has a historical museum that includes a documentary exhibit of political activities on campus before 1950. It includes a selection of photos to illustrate the leftist activities of students and staff from 1919 to 1950: the first Chinese president of the school attending a May Fourth rally in Chengdu in 1919; the campus workers' trade union in 1920; a 30 May 1925 student demonstration; a 1926 strike protesting the Wanxian incident; a 1930 anti-Christian demonstration; subsequent demonstrations against the Japanese occupation and in favour of the Communist-Guomindang United Front; and, finally, a wistful photograph of students on board a ship returning from the United States to China in October 1950. It was clearly in the university's interests to reaffirm the reversal of verdicts that declared that it was no longer the offspring of 'Enemy *Huada*' (*Huada* being the Chinese abbreviation for West China Union University), but a key medical school in the nation's plan for modernization in the 1980s.

Only twenty-five per cent of the university's students were Christians,[32] so it can be assumed that their primary motive in attending the university was to secure professional training. Most came from middle class families who could afford the tuition at a private institution, and few were political or social revolutionaries.

Students in China's Christian Colleges

Several studies of students at Christian universities in other parts of China afford the opportunity to view the West China alumni in a broader perspective. Studies of Peking Union Medical College (PUMC),[33] Yenjing,[34] and a comparative study of the thirteen Christian colleges in China[35] reveal a general trend of similarities and some specific differences between the Sichuan experience and that in other parts of the country.

The PUMC alumni are described by Mary Bullock as the second generation of Western-trained medical scientists in China. Unlike their pioneering teachers, or their counterparts in Sichuan, they had 'no need to synthesize their Confucian background with their modern education.' The PUMC campus was a relatively Westernized environment, where English predominated, and Chinese and Western professors lived in an integrated community. The parents of PUMC students were largely 'upper-class' families, including returned students, military elites, and scholar-officials. As was the case in most of the Christian colleges, very few students came from peasant families. Recruited mostly from the treaty-port provinces of coastal China,[36] the students had already been exposed to Western influence a generation before the gentry of Sichuan.[37]

The early educational background of PUMC students was similar to that of the West China students. They were recruited from missionary schools and some government schools. The difference, however, was that more than half had received a Bachelor of Science degree from Yenjing University before entering PUMC. This elite institution provided rigorous training and instruction in the English language. PUMC's curriculum could therefore build on already existing skills while WCUU had to provide basic sciences and medical English for its less sophisticated student body.

Like WCUU students, the students of PUMC aspired to study abroad. Unlike WCUU students before the influx of Eastern Chinese refugee universities, they were being groomed to be the 'medical leaders of modern China,' the professors, researchers, and administrators.[38] Although WCUU alumni eventually took their place in leadership positions in China's medical system, PUMC graduates assumed this role during the republican period, with a majority holding senior posts after graduation. By design, PUMC was geared from its inception to train a medical research and teaching elite. Its presence in West China during the Japanese occupation served to raise the standards of medical education for all the refugee medical schools in Sichuan during that period.

Like PUMC, Yenjing University in Beijing was an elite institution, populated by sophisticated students who came from affluent business families. The socioeconomic background of these students is very similar to that of WCUU students, and indeed those of all the Christian colleges in China in the 1930s. The majority of students were recruited from Yenjing's own preparatory school or from accredited Christian schools in the coastal provinces. Students were somewhat more consciously patriotic than those in other mission schools. They were dedicated to national salvation through patriotic service. The role of education was to contribute to China's modernization, and forty per cent of graduates pursued careers in education.[39]

Jessie Lutz's detailed study of the Christian colleges in China indicates the gradual shift in student background from the early scholarship students of poor Chinese Christian families to the children of affluent merchant families of the 1930s. While poor Christian parents viewed mission education as a

guarantee of future employment in the mission, later generations saw the advantage of English and science as the key to
upward mobility for their children.[40]

In the mid-1920s, a majority of student recruits had been
educated in missionary middle schools, which gave them a
background in English and sciences that government schools
and traditional schools did not offer. The graduates of government schools generally enrolled in government universities
where they would not be penalized for their insufficient English preparation. In Sichuan, students had fewer opportunities
for Western education than in the coastal provinces and cities,
which had many more Christian schools than the inland provinces. The Christian colleges in general attracted students
who wanted to study science. They offered the best facilities,
and opportunities to study abroad after graduation. By the late
1930s and early 1940s, students from government schools and
other secular middle schools began to enroll in the Christian
colleges to take advantage of a Western education.[41]

In terms of political activism, the Yenjing students had the
reputation for being the most politicized. The increasingly
centralized Guomindang government could control curriculum requirements in foreign educational institutions, but its
efforts to suppress student organizations in the 1930s were
less successful in the Christian colleges. A comparison of
campus life in the Christian colleges indicates that faculty-
student relations were based on personal contact, with a
large teacher to student ratio. Extracurricular activities
included special interest clubs and sports, and students reported many of their 'fondest memories' were inspired by
campus life.[42]

The Japanese occupation changed campus atmospheres
throughout the country. More students had to work part-time
to support themselves, especially those who were refugees in
West China. This made for a change from the traditional
intellectual disdain for manual labour,[43] and it nurtured a
certain degree of anti-elitism among the students who, separated from their families, were levelled by their wartime poverty.

The shortage of supplies and funds, the isolation of West China compared with the urban centres of East China, and the loss of libraries and laboratories abandoned in the Japanese-occupied cities led to a deterioration of morale during the war. However, the influx of sophisticated teachers and students enriched the previously secluded campus of West China Union University. On balance, the students of West China shared the same background, goals, and student life as their counterparts on other campuses, with the exception that Sichuan was more isolated from international influence, and therefore slower to respond to the changes which Western culture and education had induced in the eastern coastal cities decades earlier.

Role of Alumni in Guomindang China

The total number of WCUU medical and dental graduates by 1948 was 398 in medicine and an estimated 130 in dentistry.[44] Dr L.G. Kilborn observed in 1931, that 'We could easily place many times the number of medical and dental graduates we are able to turn out.'[45] By 1934 stringent government entrance exams attempted to restrict university enrolment to prevent a surplus of university graduates who would not be able to find employment. However, fifty per cent of WCUU students in 1934 were enrolled in medicine or dentistry, 'professions greatly in demand in this country.'[46]

The pattern of placement of graduates indicates that the original objective of the missionaries to devolve medical education to Chinese graduates was not achieved, at least not before 1949. Until 1938, when the Nationalist and provincial governments had established their health administrations in Chongqing, most medical graduates were used to staff the mission hospitals. This was in part due to the lack of Chinese hospitals and government facilities to employ these graduates. Of ten graduates in 1931, seven worked in mission hospitals.[47] As of 1938, forty-five per cent of the total 114 medical graduates and forty-seven per cent of the dental graduates were employed in mission hospitals. The rest were divided between private practice and government service, with fewer dentists recruited for the latter. Only nine per cent pursued postgraduate courses.[48] In 1934 Chiang Kai-shek personally appealed to students of the graduating class at WCUU to 'work for their country.'[49] After 1938 a significant increase in government employment of physicians occurred, with thirty-six per cent of medical graduates placed in administration or government hospitals between 1938 and 1943.[50] This shift in recruitment was due to the introduction of 'compulsory national service for new graduates,' whereby a graduate from a private university had to give one year of 'national service' to the National Health Administration.[51] In 1944 medical graduates were conscripted by the government, fifty per cent being assigned to military service, forty per cent assigned to the National Health Administration, and ten per cent allowed to defer service for one year if they taught in a university. According to Dr R.B. McClure, then a North China missionary who assessed the Guomindang's Army Medical Service, 'Army service ... is a deteriorating experience;' most conscripts were given desk jobs at the rear, and those assigned to military hospitals worked in abysmal conditions.[52]

The development of the National and Provincial Health Administrations, and the military crises of the Japanese occupation and then civil war from 1937 to 1949, introduced radical changes into the context in which the medical missionaries first conceived of medical education for China. Underlying the missionary model was the assumption that Chinese medical schools would be the first stage in the development of an indigenous system of modern medicine. The missionaries projected that their graduates would be needed to staff these schools and administer hospitals as they developed in China.

This cohort of scientific intellectuals were strategically placed to influence the succeeding generations of teachers, practitioners, and policy-makers in the medical sciences. They were poised to maintain the link between China's scientists and the international scientific community. They were first socialized in traditional China, and subsequently in a China in transformation. They were influenced by Confucian particularism, Chinese nationalism, Western liberal-democratic values, and a professional ideology stressing academic excellence and intellectual autonomy. Their education integrated liberal arts, scientific knowledge, and technical skills. The characteristics of this cohort define their predisposition to the influences that subsequently shaped their lives and careers in the People's Republic of China.

Alumni and the People's Republic of China: Birds in a Cage

It is estimated that less than half of the alumni who graduated from WCUU prior to 1949 remain in China, but those who do have played a significant role as the first post-1949 generation of teachers and researchers in the nation's effort to build a modern medical system. They are recognized for their high level of training and their academic and clinical superiority to the generations that came after them. As the first generation of post-1949 high school graduates entered the medical schools, the quality of medical graduates decreased, and the downward trend was sustained by years of anti-intellectual policy from the central government. In spite of these policies, however, the old professors, as they are called, command the respect of the younger generations. Their students, now in their fifties, are the administrators of the medical institutions. However, the teachers remain as consultants and advisers.

The hierarchy of skills in the medical field is now defined in terms of generations. The pre-1949 alumni are now largely retired and serve only in a consultative role. The 1950s generation are skilled clinicians who filled the administrative void left by the older generation until the mid-1980s. The 1960s graduates are the attending physicians and have the least training. They began to take over administrative leadership in the mid-1980s. The 1970s generation is non-existent professionally. The 1980s generation has reportedly surpassed its teachers; the elite of this group have gone abroad to study, and as was the case with their predecessors in the 1940s, many have not returned. If the lesson of the old generation's Sisyphean career path is a message to them, they are not likely to return until the intellectual climate is more hospitable.

For those who stayed, their professional lives careened back and forth with the changes in China's political winds. What remained stable, in spite of the policy upheavals in medical care and education, was the basic core of values and beliefs inculcated in the alumni during their early careers. The factors that influenced the formation of attitudes and career paths of the medical and dental alumni of West China Union University were their socioeconomic background, their individual motivations, and their educational experiences. These factors affected the way the alumni responded to the external stimuli of political and cultural forces. The impact of the Anti-Japanese War, the introduction of a foreign educational model, knowledge, and technology, and the political instability of China during the formative years of the lives of the alumni all contributed to a composite pattern of beliefs, attitudes, and behaviours that characterized this cohort of scientific intellectuals. We have noted that as a group, they tended to be conservative and pragmatic. However, they were also exposed to Western culture, which they integrated with their earlier socialization in China's traditional cultural norms. They were taught to 'roll between two cultures,' as one of their foreign professors used to advise them.[1]

In 1949 many of the alumni were characterized by a deep sense of patriotism, motivating those who were still in China as well as those who made the arduous journey home from study abroad, in the early 1950s, to contribute to China's self-strengthening. They were also committed to the Western model of scientific medical education in a comprehensive university, where arts and sciences coexisted, and clinical medicine had its base in a strong scientific foundation. Furthermore, they believed in the standards of excellence set by their professors, both in China and abroad, and were dedicated to the concept of an elite medical corps that set the standards for education and care. In terms of their professional values, they maintained their goal of professional autonomy, and they had been taught medical ethics exemplified by the tenets of Christian humanitarianism and the Hippocratic Oath. This bound them to a code of conduct that required them to offer medical care to anyone who required it and to adhere to their professional standards before all else.

It was with this disposition that the alumni entered the era of Communist rule in China. This chapter examines the career paths of the alumni, including their professional role and their political histories from 1949 to 1989. It also looks at the changing role of the medical school during this period and of medical and dental professionals within the ranks of China's scientific elite.

The Transition to Communism

In the autumn of 1949 the Chinese Communists consolidated control of most of the country, including Sichuan, and began to transform the institutional structures of Guomindang China. Their agenda included the logistics of political control, the introduction of new institutional structures and educational models, and the resocialization of the intellectual elite as well as of the 'masses.' This intellectual elite, the bearers of ideas and traditions, had long been regarded by China's ruling elite as a key element in establishing and maintaining political power. Therefore, one of the primary targets for radical change in the New China was the system of education, considered a crucial element in political control.

The university began to feel the effects of government policy by the spring of 1950. Curricular reform was the first stage, with the introduction of Marxist-Leninist courses in philosophy, economics, and history, and the exclusion of courses in ethics and religion. Dr Kilborn observed that the Christian principle underlying Western medical ethics, based on equal access to medical care, was unacceptable to the Communist principle of clearly defining enemies and friends based on socioeconomic status. Foreign missionaries and

Chinese doctors alike were criticized by Communist cadres for offering medical care to class enemies.

Mass meetings became a frequent part of campus life, as the Communist Party officials worked assiduously to inculcate the new ideology in the minds of students and faculty. Some faculty members were singled out for criticism in mass meetings, accused of harbouring reactionary views which hampered the development of revolutionary China. Governance of the university was temporarily 'democratized,' as students and workers were added to college councils, in some cases outnumbering faculty members.[2]

Although foreign missionary faculty who remained in China after 1949 were initially allowed to continue their work, they were increasingly isolated from their Chinese colleagues and restricted in their influence on the university. The imposition of high taxes on missionary institutions added to the strained relations between the Chinese Christian institutions and their home boards, who were loath to pay from already depleted wartime resources and wary of the uncertain future of religious and institutional freedom under the newly established Communist government. But while most of the missionary hospitals and schools were closed or taken over by local government, the university continued to function.

Missionaries who elected to remain at their posts in Chengdu were caught by an upsurge of anti-foreign sentiment after the outbreak of the Korean War in 1950. Government uneasiness about the presence of foreign nationals when the country was at war led to increasing isolation of and hostility against the missionaries. As well as in suspicion of missionaries and their Chinese associates as potential enemy spies, the anti-foreign movement manifested itself in the rejection of English as the language of instruction in the medical college, and in an escalation of attacks in the press and mass meetings against the imperialist aggression of Christian evangelism in China.

Chinese professors and students began to avoid the foreign missionaries for fear of reprisals by the Communist cadres who now controlled the university's administration. Individual

Chinese faculty were pressured to criticize their foreign colleagues in public denunciations of American imperialism. As
Dr Leslie Kilborn, the dean of the Medical College, reported,
the State Administrative Council issued an order in December
1950 which linked medical missionary work with imperialist
aggression. The edict, reported and translated by Kilborn, read
as follows: 'For more than one hundred years now American
Imperialism has not only committed political, financial and
military aggression, she has emphasized even more acts of
cultural aggression over a long period. The most important
thing about this type of cultural aggression is that it puts out
large amounts of money to support religious, educational,
cultural, medical, literary and relief work, etc. and uses the
above agencies to forward deception, doping, and the instilling
of slavish thoughts, so seeking the spiritual angle to enslave
the Chinese people.'[3]

The university archives contained ample evidence of relations between former governments and the university administration, and these files were used in assembling the case
against *Wei Huada*, 'Unconstitutional (illegal) West China
Union University.'[4] During the 1920s and 1930s, warlords and
municipal officials frequently requested, as a special favour,
the admission of one of their relatives to medical school;
Deng Xi-hou and Liu Wen-hui were among the warlords who
had corresponded with the university. During the 1930s, when
the Guomindang government demanded that all missionary
and foreign schools register with the Ministry of Education,
the president of WCUU sought elite support for the institution.
Dr Zhang Lin-gao (Lincoln Dsang) invited the Governor of
Sichuan to chair the board of directors in 1933, and he frequently asked military leaders to address the graduating class.
Financial aid to the school was forthcoming from Chengdu's
ruling elite, who were also helpful in placing graduates in
jobs. In 1949, only months before the Communist take-over,
high-level Guomindang officials and members of the gentry
attended the celebration of WCUU's thirty-ninth anniversary.
At the same time, President Zhang criticized the excesses of
the Guomindang Youth Corps in harassing left-wing students

and called for developing links with the community in accordance with their needs. The speeches stressed the need to combine new ideas with the old traditions of WCUU, in particular the values of Christian humanitarianism, mutual respect, and community cooperation.[5] A long history of association with the former government, however, could not be undone by a sudden shift to conciliation with the new regime. The Communists systematically rooted out any potential threats to their system and its claim to moral and political authority. Zhang Lin-gao and other members of the former administration were arrested in 1950.[6]

By 4 January 1951, several days after the State Council meeting, West China Union University was nationalized, and a military control commission took charge of the administration. Thence began a reorganization of the university along the lines of the Soviet model of specialized institutions. The university was gradually dismantled, beginning with the abolition of the School of Theology. The College of Dentistry and Medicine was formally separated into two institutions. The curriculum for both courses was shortened to five years from the original seven, in line with the policy of meeting the country's short-term health-care needs. A two-and-a-half year course was introduced to train several hundred paramedics. In addition to their regular teaching responsibilities, medical faculty were expected to teach in the short course, as well as in the military medical school and a municipal health workers school. They also had clinical responsibilities, and as foreign-trained specialists in Western medicine, they were requested to provide medical care to senior government officials throughout the country.[7] The added work-load combined with political indoctrination meetings led to exhaustion of the overburdened staff and a decline in the quality of teaching and care.

As 1951 progressed, government fear of counter-revolutionary activity increased. Arrests and executions, some part of the movement for land reform and some part of the 'resist America, aid Korea' war effort, escalated. Senior faculty, particularly Christians, and some missionary faculty, were arrested as spies and counter-revolutionaries. The first graduate of WCUU, Dr Liu Yue-tin (*sic*), was executed in Rongxian. The reports of arrests and executions continued, as a reign of terror replaced the Chinese Communists' earlier moderation. Kilborn recounted the cases of several of his Chinese colleagues and students who were forced to denounce foreign missionaries. Many responded by criticizing deceased missionaries, until authorities discovered this and demanded that accusations be directed at those still present in Chengdu.

In spite of the increasing anti-foreign hostility, the government requested five of the mission families to remain at the university in their teaching or administrative positions. At the same time, Chinese faculty and senior administrators were either arrested or sent to 're-education camps' for political indoctrination. A concerted effort was made to remove every vestige of foreign influence in the university, including the removal of foreign names from buildings. Kilborn described the systematic elimination of English signs from the campus, from the 'Letters' plate over the staff mailboxes, to a sign over the entrance to Hart College that read 'The Truth Shall Make You Free.' Apparently, a Greek motto reading 'You Shall Know the Truth,' at the entrance to the medical college, was overlooked by the authorities, prompting the disheartened Dr Kilborn to write, 'May it long remain and be prophetic of the future when the truth will be known.'

Kilborn, along with the few remaining Western faculty, saw the gradual dismantling of their efforts of the previous forty years. Not only was the curriculum truncated, and faculty overextended to the point of exhaustion, but by 1952 all English medical textbooks were banned and replaced with mass-produced, poor-quality Chinese substitutes which were hurriedly prepared to fill the gap. By March 1952 the missionaries had left Chengdu for the safety of Hong Kong. Their contacts with their Chinese colleagues dwindled until they were extinguished for almost a quarter of a century, as contact with foreigners became politically dangerous in a climate of anti-Western hostility.

In the early years of Communist rule, Soviet orthodoxy replaced Western science in the universities and research institutes all over the country. Scientists were expected to learn Russian rather than English; Soviet experts replaced North American and European faculty as senior advisers in the universities; and Soviet scientific models were imposed on Western-trained Chinese researchers and clinicians. Western imperialism was blamed for holding back the development of indigenous capacity in Chinese science, medicine, and economic development. The Soviet organization of educational institutions influenced the 'realignment of specialties' (yuanxitiaozheng) that occurred in 1952. The professional schools of the university were reorganized as separate institutions, and the medical college, which included the schools of medicine, dentistry, pharmacy, and public health, was renamed Sichuan Medical College. The arts and science faculty was transferred to Sichuan University, located on another campus. Thus began the isolation of the medical sciences not only from Western influence, but also from the influence of any other disciplines at the university.

Alumni Career Patterns

By this time, most of the alumni from other parts of China had either returned home or left China. It is estimated that half of the medical, dental, and pharmacy graduates emigrated shortly before or after 1949 to Hong Kong, the United States, Canada, and Western Europe. Of those who remained in China, the majority returned to their prewar alma maters (before they sought wartime refuge on the campus of WCUU). The PUMC students returned to Beijing, Tianjin students to Tianjin, and so on for Shanghai, Guangzhou, and other cities in China. Most of the refugee students who remained in Sichuan found positions on the university faculty.

As a group, the alumni occupied leadership positions in Chinese medical and dental institutions, including hospitals, schools, and research institutes. They formed the senior ranks of medical professionals in the country, with the longest

duration of training and standardized education in the skills
and knowledge of Western medicine. More than two-thirds of
the alumni occupied academic positions throughout the country, serving as professors and, department heads, and increasingly after 1989, as semi-retired senior advisers in China's medical schools. This group is represented in the leading medical
schools in the country, including PUMC, Shanghai Medical College, Zhongshan Medical College, and Sichuan Medical College.
The second-largest group entered clinical practice, often as
department heads or senior administrators in urban, provincial, or county hospitals. This group, as they age, are also joining the ranks of a senior advisory system in the hospital administration. A much smaller number entered government or
military service. Although the alumni were granted formal
recognition, their real authority was limited by the authority
of the Chinese Communist Party.[8] The party did acknowledge, however, that Western medical education had a place in
China's medical modernization.

The alumni of the College of Dentistry are perhaps among
the best-known WCUU alumni in China outside of Sichuan.
They formed the nuclei of university dental faculties, and
trained the next generations of dental scientists and clinicians. It is widely acknowledged that WCUU was the birth-
place of modern dentistry in China, and it was in fact a recognized centre of excellence in both Guomindang and, later,
Communist China.

The data on career patterns of the pharmacy graduates are
incomplete, with data available for only the 1923–45 period.
One can approximate their career profiles from this information, which indicates that about twenty-five per cent of
them worked in production or retail units, 16.5 per cent
worked in clinical jobs, and fifteen per cent worked in academic positions. Of the 127 alumni for whom there are data,
seventeen joined the faculty of the university in Chengdu.
Two alumni who left China in 1949 work in research and
clinical pharmacy respectively. Although records for the
pharmacy graduates are not available, it is interesting to note
that 1980s Chinese statistical data on human resources in

higher education aggregates medical and pharmacy institutions and personnel.

The medical curriculum prior to 1949 consisted of a seven-year course, with two years in premedical sciences (which dental students were also required to complete). In 1950, the curriculum was shortened to six years, in the effort to provide basic health care to a burgeoning population. Short courses of three to four years duration were also introduced into some medical schools. The Soviet model of training various levels of medical personnel to deliver preventive and primary care was adopted, and the training of an elite who were dedicated to tertiary care in urban centres was decreased. In 1954 the residency (postgraduate) trainings programs were replaced by political rather than clinical training. In 1959 the curriculum was further shortened to five years. The universities closed during the Cultural Revolution, and when medical schools re-opened (in the case of Sichuan Medical College, this was not until 1978), some schools established a five year course with one year of internship. However, there has been no standard duration of medical training adopted by all medical schools. The length of training varies widely among institutions, and from year to year, since 1950. This has resulted in an imprecise definition of medical professionals: there are numerous grades of doctors, dentists, and pharmacists, depending on the prevailing educational policy and institution. This fluctuation in standards has placed the pre-1949 alumni at the highest level of expertise in terms of medical education within China.

Political Careers

In an anti-Western, anti-intellectual, and anti-elitist political climate, the alumni of WCUU and other missionary universities were ready targets for political attack. They were initially singled out for re-education in the early 1950s, as the Communist leadership sought to eradicate the bourgeois imperialist influence of their Western educators. Western-trained intellectuals were sent for Marxist re-education before they were allowed to influence the succeeding generations of Chi-

nese university students. Although few medical and dental
students were politically active or even interested during their
student days, even the minority who were involved in underground Communist activities were tainted by their Western
education. Almost a third of the alumni surveyed for this
study had spent time at North American or British universities and thus had the further handicap of foreign contacts
outside the country. This was particularly difficult during the
Korean War period, when foreign association could lead to
suspicion of espionage, but few of the alumni were accused of
serious crimes against the state.

The anti-Rightist campaign of 1957 posed a new threat to
medical alumni, as the medical colleges were assigned a quota
of individuals to fill the roster of accused Rightists. In the
case of Sichuan Medical College, the quota was three to five
per cent. When it appeared that ten per cent of the graduating
class of 1957 were under attack, the campaign was relaxed
because physicians were required for clinical service. Only
two of the survey respondents were labelled as Rightists, both
of them women alumnae who had graduated in the 1930s.[9] It
appears that an initial spate of labels, which decimated the
ranks of medical clinicians, was reversed when it was discovered that good doctors were in short supply. The attacks
were deflected away from clinicians towards more dispensable
faculty members, for example, English and humanities
teachers.

The Great Leap Forward campaign of 1958–9 served to di-
lute further the effectiveness of the scientific elite by imposing short-term educational goals in a mass effort to provide
preventive and primary health care for the whole population.
Research and teaching programs designed to achieve longer-
term objectives were obliterated and replaced by short-term
courses and politically motivated applied research. However,
the economic failure generated by Great Leap directives led to
a retrenchment of earlier policies, and in 1961 education and
research briefly resumed their pre-1958 focus.

While the anti-rightist campaign, in terms of the scientific
community, was tinged with a modicum of pragmatism, the

Cultural Revolution was nihilistic in the extreme. During 1966–72, many intellectuals were killed or driven to suicide. Universities were closed for up to six years, and the entire system of research and higher education was virtually destroyed. Labelled the 'ninth stinking category,' – the 'cows, ghosts, snakes, and monsters' fouling the political landscape of revolutionary China – the old intellectuals became social pariahs.

Of the alumni who responded to questions about their experiences during the Cultural Revolution, many judged that their treatment had been moderately severe compared with that of their colleagues, considering that they were still alive. Only four respondents considered their persecution to be minimal. One of these worked in an area that was highlighted as a policy priority by Party Chairman Mao Zedong, and the other worked directly for the Chairman as his personal physician. More than half of the alumni surveyed reported moderate to moderately severe treatment, ranging from confinement for up to one year, confiscation of their medical texts and journals, public humiliation and forced self-criticism sessions, and banishment from their teaching or clinical positions. Some continued to work at menial jobs, as orderlies or ward clerks, while others were exiled to rural areas to provide primary health care or to train 'barefoot' doctors. Most reported that they were still consulted by junior colleagues and patients on difficult medical problems, and they continued to provide care from their demoted positions. In some cases, high-level leaders who required sophisticated medical diagnosis or treatment called these doctors out of exile for a brief period, so that they could provide their services.

One-third of this group who were survivors of the upheaval of the Cultural Revolution reported severe maltreatment. They were subjected to physical torture and long-term confinement and isolation. The treatment of the intellectual elite throughout the country was similar to that reported by the WCUU alumni.[10] However, the individuals who received the worst treatment were more likely to be second-generation intellectuals (that is, their parents were also graduates of elite institutions) who were in leadership positions. The severity of the struggle also tended to vary among different work units, and from region to region in the country. In Sichuan, county towns reportedly experienced more violent political struggles than the cities. Alumni at PUMC in Beijing were subjected to harsher treatment than the majority of their colleagues in Chengdu. Many survivors, both alumni and their students, reported that their children were traumatized by the spectacle of their parents being forced to crawl down the streets of Chengdu wearing dunce caps or forced to jump from high walls as they were publicly denounced for their counter-revolutionary crimes as bourgeois academics. The senior teachers at Sichuan Medical College were locked into one of the teaching buildings, made to sleep next to the anatomy laboratory cadavers, and forced to write confessions of their political crimes. After varying lengths of time, most of them were 'sent down' to the rural autonomous prefecture of Liangshan, about 200 kilometres southwest of Chengdu. Separated from their families, they worked in the countryside as medics or labourers for months or years, until the end of the Cultural Revolution. Furthermore, their children were barred from educational opportunities. These were reserved for the children of workers, peasants, and soldiers, who were considered more 'politically correct' than the privileged offspring of urban intellectuals. While the alumni themselves were rehabilitated following the Cultural Revolution, many of their children continue to work in manual or low-level jobs.

The university remained closed for eight years, from 1966 to 1973. In 1973, a three-year medical curriculum was introduced, and when the old professors returned in 1978, the short-course students returned for further training. Some of these students won scholarships to study abroad, and others entered postgraduate training under the tutelage of the old professors.

Except for those who retired because of advanced age or ill-health, all the surviving alumni were restored to their former positions by 1978, and most were promoted. Only six were returned to their posts by 1972, another one in each of 1973 and 1974, and the rest in 1978, when those senior intellectuals who had been exiled to the countryside returned to the cities. Under the auspices of the Ministries of Finance and Public Health, the old intellectuals were re-assimilated into their former positions, requested to resume teaching, and awarded salary increases.

Role of Alumni in China's Medical System

Studies of China's achievements in higher education, published in the 1980s, provide some perspective on the role of the pre-1949 alumni in post-1949 China. Even before 1949, they were an elite in terms of numbers. This cohort, born between 1904 and 1929, belonged to a group of university graduates that totalled about 40,000 throughout the entire country. This includes graduates born before 1929 and represents all disciplines.[11] Analysts of China's statistics on education cite the abnormal age distribution of academic staff as a problem in human resource development. This is most noticeable at the senior level, where, in 1983, when graduate training was moving into high gear, there were no full professors under forty years of age, and the majority (3,895 out of a total of 4,472, or eighty-seven per cent) were over sixty years of age.[12] The largest number of graduates were born between 1935 and 1946, but the subsequent generation, born between 1947 and 1954, produced the smallest number of graduates because of the political upheavals and the destruction of the education system during the years when they would have attended university. The system of promotion exacerbated this distribution, since academic rank was based on a combination of political and professional criteria, and was abolished altogether in 1972. When it was restored in 1978, many professors of the pre-1949 generations, whose rank had been frozen for almost two decades, were promoted to full professor. The oldest cohort, the pre-1949 graduates, have had to serve through the period when, in the normal course of events, a younger generation should have been in place to take over from them.

Numerically, the pre-1949 cohort is a small fraction of the
total medical personnel in China. There were only 9,000
graduates of medicine and pharmacy from 1928 to 1947.[13]
From 1949 to 1983 the numbers increased more than fifty-fold
to 496,600. The number of postgraduates is even more rari-
fied, with only six students recorded as enrolled in postgraduate study in 1947, eighty-three in 1949, and thirty-two in
1950. Between 1951 and 1966, there was a stable enrolment
of about 250 graduate students each year. After universities
reopened in 1978, enrolment jumped to 1,474, and the next
year to 3,113. The data show that there were only 2,288 full
professors in all faculties in Chinese universities in 1977 (1.2
per cent of the total faculty), thus placing the WCUU cohort in
a key position in rebuilding the graduate training programs
until sufficient numbers of faculty could be upgraded. Another
factor contributing to the small number of senior teaching
faculty was the incidence of illness among those faculty returning from a period of exile in remote regions of China or
those recovering from physical and mental abuse perpetrated
during the Cultural Revolution. In 1977, 10.5 per cent of
China's higher education faculty did not teach, owing to illness. Moreover, many of those who did return were dedicated
to restoring the nation's research capacity, and about one-
third of this senior echelon were assigned to research work.[14]
In 1977 university entrance examinations were re-introduced,
and a new generation of highly qualified students entered the
medical schools in 1978.

The critical role of the senior faculty was reinforced in
1982, when the Twelfth National Congress of the Communist
Party placed education and science among the top priorities
for national development. Symbolic of the party's support for
the scientific elite, commemorative postage stamps of senior
scientists who had served in the Chinese Communist Party
began to appear in the early 1980s. They lauded the achievements of those who had received a Western education before
1949 and who continued to contribute to China's scientific
development after that time.[15] In 1987, the *People's Daily*
published a glowing obituary in memory of Zhang Xiao-qian,

a graduate of Yale-in-China, Johns Hopkins and Stanford universities who had served on the faculty of PUMC. He was eulogized as a 'giant star and pioneer of Western medicine in China,'[16] and Deng Xiaoping, President Li Xiannian, and Chen Yun were among the political elite who contributed wreaths to the memorial ceremonies. The message to China's elder intellectual elite was clear: they were no longer pariahs in the New China, but a revered group on whom the new drive for scientific modernization relied to rebuild its foundation. Furthermore, the party, as it had done in the early 1950s, attempted to attract the scientific elite to its ranks and thus strengthen their loyalty to the regime's policies.

In 1989 the *China Daily* published an article about the memoirs of Dr C.C. Chen, well-known as one of the pioneers of public-health research and policy in pre-revolutionary China. Chen, who had been hounded politically for most of his career after 1949, was acknowledged as an inspiring teacher and contributor to the rural health of China, and an example of the fruits of the cross-cultural transfer which took place more than a half century earlier, when Chen graduated from PUMC and worked with his teacher, Dr John B. Grant, to develop a model of rural health care at the famous Dingxian experimental community.[17] The Chinese scholars who had received training from Western educators and institutions, and attempted to adapt this knowledge to build China's scientific and educational foundation, were, in the 1980s, finally granted some recognition for their contribution and worth in China's drive towards modernization.

With the announcement of the Open-Door policy, the government encouraged links with foreign sources of science, technology, and financial investment. Many of those in teaching institutions were called on to re-establish links with their foreign professors from the 1930s and 1940s. These Western-educated alumni had English language skills, an understanding of Western culture, and links with foreign institutions that predated the Communist period. Although it was the 1950s generation who now administered medical institutions and held leadership positions in the universities and hospitals, the older generations were instrumental in establishing institutional links with universities and research institutes in Europe, North America, and Japan. Considerably more cosmopolitan than their younger colleagues who had never been outside China or had studied in Soviet bloc countries, they were the new vanguard in the effort to internationalize China's science and technology.

When the senior faculty returned to the campus of Sichuan Medical College in 1978, they were invited to form a consultative committee (*Zixun weiyuanhui*) to advise the administration on policy matters. This committee operated for eight years, from 1980 to 1988. Its role was to assist in setting goals for educational reform, participate in the investigation and evaluation committee for the promotion of junior faculty, and direct post-graduate research. In the area of educational policy, it addressed the issues of curricular reform, scientific research, medical services, and the university's international relations. Although the party dominated policy, and the central Ministry of Public Health set the guidelines for educational policy, local units decided on implementation plans. Furthermore, there was some opportunity to respond to central policy initiatives, through the Chinese People's Political Consultative Conference (CPPCC). This body of senior intellectuals, often outside the Chinese Communist Party but increasingly made up of retired Communist Party members, has no real political power but serves in an advisory capacity and has the authority of its members' seniority and achievements. Six of the senior alumni from Chengdu were appointed to this committee, and other faculty members served on the provincial and municipal branches of the CPPCC, and on the provincial People's Congress, the provincial arm of the central government.

The senior alumni also actively pursued the restoration of international links for the medical college. They began to assemble a list of alumni throughout China and overseas and to contact foreign professors. Dr Cao Zhongliang, who had been the first Chinese Dean of Medicine before 1949, reestablished the alumni association, and with his son, Dr Cao

Zeyi, President of the College, and Dr C.C. Chen, established institutional links with the University of Toronto Faculty of Medicine, the alma mater of many of the missionaries who had helped to establish the university before 1949. The medical college also established relations with the University of Washington in Seattle and Tulane University Medical School in New Orleans. With the approach of the university's seventy-fifth anniversary in 1985, plans were made to organize a reunion of faculty and alumni. The name of the college was changed to West China University of Medical Sciences (WCUMS), reflecting its historical roots. The link with the University of Toronto, and an active alumni association in Hong Kong, provided valuable resources in the effort to upgrade the quality of education and research at the university. This trend was common throughout China, as universities sought to re-establish international links.

WCUMS is one of six key medical schools among the 112 schools in the country. It is directly under the control of the Ministries of Education and Public Health in Beijing. The premier school in China is Beijing Union Medical College (formerly a Rockefeller Foundation school, PUMC), which has an eight-year curriculum designed to train a medical science elite. The other key schools have a six-year course. WCUMS is among the third rank of the key schools, after Beijing and Shanghai, but it is the leading tertiary-care institution in West China, serving a population of 100 million, and it is the centre of medical education in the province of Sichuan. The senior alumni, along with the administration, developed a proposal to increase the medical curriculum at the key schools to seven years, using WCUMS as a model to test the policy. The new curriculum included medical ethics, psychology, literature, and history, in addition to the basic sciences, standard medical curriculum, and clinical training. This proposal was adopted in 1989, and thirty students are annually enrolled in this course. At the same time, WCUMS offers postgraduate medical education, as well as the standard five-year course and a three-year course for rural physicians.

Views on Medical Modernization

An examination of the views of alumni on medical modernization reveals a similarity of ideas among this cohort. Those
who responded to the survey were almost unanimous in their
recommendation that international exchange was an essential
component of the modernization process. The second most
important step in upgrading China's medical resources was
the elevation of educational standards; this was promoted
with the adoption of university entrance examinations in
1977. There was also general agreement that medical education would benefit from interdisciplinary studies, and the
notion of a return to the comprehensive university model was
raised. An emphasis on basic sciences and research was
stressed by more than half of the alumni who responded to
this question in the survey. Few respondents advocated less
political intervention in medical education. This may be
owing to a deeply ingrained reluctance to discuss political
issues. Technological upgrading was also mentioned by only
a small number of alumni. Several respondents explained that
in fact expensive technology was not a first priority in medical modernization, considering China's current stage of development. The need to foster independent thinking in place of
didactic pedagogy was raised by only five of the respondents.
This contrasts with the views of the 1960s generation of
alumni and also a report by the World Bank on China's health
care system,[18] which stressed the need to develop problem-
solving skills and autonomy among medical students, rather
than rote learning and unquestioning adherence to established
practices.

The medical policies that dominated the early period of
communist rule, and the subsequent periods of 'radical' policy
during the Great Leap Forward and the Cultural Revolution,
included an emphasis on the development of traditional Chinese medicine and on preventive health care. The success of
these policies, which made use of China's scarce resources in
the most economical manner for rapid progress in health care,
greatly influenced other Third World health development

policies, and indeed they became a model for the World Health Organization in the early 1970s. However, considering the priorities for medical modernization in the late 1980s, only four alumni supported the notion that there should be further emphasis on the development of traditional Chinese medicine, and only two cited prevention as an important aspect of medical education. The report by the World Bank raises issues similar to those raised by the majority of alumni: inadequate training in basic sciences, weak graduate programs, and the inappropriateness of high technology as a priority in the improvement of medical education.[19]

As the senior alumni were increasingly drawn back into the mainstream of medical development from 1978 on, they were part of an overall policy to recruit an alienated intelligentsia to the cause of China's modernization. This cohort, the members of which were motivated at several stages in their careers by a deep sense of patriotism, once again responded to the need and made their contribution to rebuilding international scientific links and the medical care and education system. In a nationwide attempt to recognize the value of intellectual work, the Chinese Communist Party opened its membership to senior intellectuals and acknowledged the right of the 'democratic' political parties to exist. There is still a great reluctance among the intellectual elite to disclose political stance; however half of the alumni responded that they belonged to a political party, and of these, thirty per cent belonged to the Communist Party.[20] The September Third Party, an organization of scientists and engineers that was initiated in the 1940s, was listed by twelve per cent of respondents. Thirty-four per cent of respondents claimed no political affiliation, and sixteen per cent did not respond to the question. Considering the apolitical nature of this group during their student days, there is a relatively high incidence of participation in political organizations. In addition to party membership, ten of the alumni serve on government committees, one on the Central Committee, and the rest on the Chinese People's Political Consultative Conference and local people's congresses.

Networks

In most political systems, the scientific elite form a network, which may exert political influence in the realm of science and educational policy, or simply serve as an expanded peer group in the development of research and teaching, and the allocation of personnel. These functions were monopolized by a centralized state in the early 1950s. The anti-intellectual policy winds of the ensuing thirty years, and the complete ostracization of China's medical elite during the Cultural Revolution, made it impossible to maintain a network among the alumni of WCUU, other than the ongoing association of those working at the same institution. They lost contact with their peers in other parts of China who had returned home from their refuge in Chengdu after the Sino-Japanese War. With the closing of China's borders in 1950 they lost contact with their peers who had emigrated overseas. The tradition of staying at one institution for one's entire career further reinforced the isolation of alumni, in spite of the fact that the alumni association was not formally abolished until the Cultural Revolution.

The alumni associations of the thirteen former Protestant colleges in China continued to thrive in Hong Kong. They sponsored social activities, social welfare systems, and a reinforcement of the values they had learned as students, expressed by their school songs, and by mottoes which were proudly displayed at annual gatherings. The WCUU Alumni Association in Hong Kong played a particularly important role in re-establishing a liaison with its alma mater in 1985 and thereafter. Under the strong leadership of Dr Denny Huang and his wife, Esther Huang, both alumni of the university, the association hosts visiting scholars from Chengdu and provides scholarships, equipment, and supplies for the campus in Chengdu.

Dr Cao Zhongliang revived the alumni association in Chengdu, reaching out to the branch in Hong Kong, to individuals overseas, and to newly established branches in China. The Beijing branch, led by Dr Wu Wei-ran, has a membership of

700, including graduates from the 1920s to the present. They publish a monthly newsletter, host visiting professors from Chengdu, and hold several social activities each year. The association in Chengdu began to publish a bulletin in October 1985, which highlights the accomplishments of graduates, reviews the international links of the WCUMS, and recounts historical vignettes of the university's early days. This seems rather insignificant from a Western perspective, but in a political system that so clearly demarcates pre-liberation and post-liberation history, any institution established before the revolution of 1949 was suspect, and Sichuan Medical College's early history was virtually obliterated in the movement to change alumni alliances, values, and beliefs. In spite of this ideological blockade, the alumni remained a critical link in the development of medical education and care, through their students and, eventually, through their re-emergence during the Open-Door period from 1982 to 1989.

From Pariah to 'Backbone': The Changing Role of Western-Trained Intellectuals

There are many ways to approach an assessment of the role of a Western-trained scientific elite in China's medical modernization. From the missionary perspective, one might focus on the failures and successes of their model to transform China's medical system. From a generational perspective, one can focus on their socialization and the resulting beliefs, values, and attitudes that characterize this group. From the broader perspective of Chinese society, one can focus on the role of modernizing elites, and place a modernizing medical elite within this context. Finally, an international and historical perspective focuses on the limits of cross-cultural technology transfer.

Successes and Failures

When Omar Kilborn left southern Ontario for the remoteness of West China, his intention was to evangelize the population of Sichuan and provide medical care for the missionaries. Within a short time of arriving, Kilborn began to see the role that modern medicine could play in improving the physical and spiritual well-being of China. From the early days of medical evangelization, he began to develop a model for enhancing the efficiency of his efforts. Gradually, the call to medical missionaries to 'multiply themselves' grew into a full-scale university medical college, dedicated to training physicians, dentists, and pharmacists to the standards of the Western medical professions.

An assessment of the achievements of the College of Medicine and Dentistry in 1949 would conclude that its elitist approach to medical modernization failed to meet China's desperate need for medical care by mid-century. The West China Union University model was based on the notion that the provision of tertiary-care institutions and research-oriented medical education would provide a basis on which to build a modern medical system. The elites thus trained would train the future generations of China's medical profession from their urban, scientifically based medical university. From the practical viewpoint of China's Communist policy-makers in 1950, training a small medical elite was irrelevant to the country's immediate requirements for public sanitation and primary health care. The WCUU trained only 808 medical science graduates between 1920 and 1950, to serve a population of over sixty million in Sichuan Province. Numerically, they were insignificant in the rapid transformation of the 'the sick man of Asia,' as China was known in the first half of the twentieth century.

In spite of its failure by the time missionary involvement in China's medical modernization ended, the notion of training an elite with assistance from the most scientifically advanced nations has persisted both in China and in the rest of the developing world. For a decade after the missionaries left, the Soviet Union provided the expertise, technology, and ethos for transforming China into a prosperous industrialized nation. Following the autarkic period of xenophobic self-reliance under Mao's increasingly radical policies, China once again opened her doors in 1978 to foreign influence and assistance. However, the clash of values inherent in technological change and transfer from another culture continues to plague this process. There continues to be a tension between the technology and accompanying value systems of the West and those of Chinese society.

At the time the missionaries attempted 'to make over a me-

dieval society in terms of modern knowledge,'[1] they believed
that the transfer of modern knowledge would lead to modern-
ization only if accompanied by Christian beliefs and values.
Their disappointment with the failure of Christianity in
China rationalized their disillusionment with the rejection of
Western medical education by the Chinese Communists.

The failure to transmit their values and ideas from West to
East lay not so much in the failure of the Chinese to accept
them, as in the obstacles to integrating new ideas into the
prevailing system. Cross-cultural communication was understood by some missionaries at the time, and by some of their
Chinese students, who were encouraged to 'roll between two
cultures.'[2] With the missionaries setting the agenda for medical modernization, however, the result was a 'cultural fragmentation' of their students. Trained by professors who
believed in professional autonomy and liberal individualism,
these graduates had to integrate their liberal university education with the realities of a Confucian culture in which individuals were subordinate to society.

The attitudinal context of the transfer of knowledge in this
case also created the challenge of operating within the political context of the recipient society. The missionaries recognized the need to couple political resolve with modern
technology to achieve development.[3] They recognized the
importance of identifying local political elites who would
expedite the delivery of their message and services to the
population. The administrators of the medical and dental
college in Chengdu were always conscious of the need to
operate with the approval and support of prevailing political
forces, be they warlord generals in Sichuan, Nationalist government ministers, or Communist cadres. In addition to co-
opting support, missionaries believed that physical prosperity
and development would lead to a more stable political order
and, by extension, a more peaceful and equitable world order.
The Social Gospel that motivated the Canadian 'evangelists
of science' professed the belief in integrating 'ultimate human
goals in the social, economic and political order.'[4] As Sichuan
became more integrated into the Chinese political system

after the warlord period, the missionaries, who now could at least identify the government they were trying to influence, were frustrated by an increasing sense of Chinese nationalism and the concomitant independence of China from foreign control.

The combination of missionary goals and Chinese expectations and responses led to other problems of cross-cultural interaction. Aware of the possibility that attending a foreign-run Christian university could be socially disruptive, university educators at WCUU deliberately provided student accommodation which would not develop 'a habit and a style of living beyond what they would be able to command after leaving college.'[5] Many graduates who were sponsored to study abroad never returned after the 1949 revolution. Many were unwilling to face the hardships and uncertainties that awaited them in China.

The Western model of institutionalized medical care provides a further example of the social implications of cross-cultural transfer. Maternity care in mission hospitals required that women deliver their infants in a hospital, according to the prevailing practice in North American obstetrics. This led to serious consequences for women who complied; they had to face the traditional 'threshold' laws, which forbade women to cross the entrance to their homes for thirty days after child-birth. The best obstetrical technical care had difficulty competing with the limitations of entrenched social custom.[6]

The principle of equitable access to medical care further challenged traditional Chinese values. Missionary doctors were committed to providing care for the sick regardless of political or religious persuasion. Chinese loyalties were more particularistic, based on family, clan, or other group associations. The notion of equal treatment was alien in this setting. In the early days of the West China Mission, the local populace took advantage of the neutrality of mission compounds, where wounded soldiers from opposing warlord armies could find refuge, and fleeing civilians could seek protection.

The foreign agents of change could introduce new knowledge, techniques, and values, but they had no power to con-

trol their integration into the social and political system of
the host society. They had no power to assure the means of
social change or the equitability of the distribution of the
benefits of their technology. In retrospect, their only course of
action was to transfer technology and knowledge to an elite
who would then be responsible for translating and diffusing it
within their own society.

The medical missionaries were involved in an ongoing
debate about the most effective strategy for long-term change.
Some argued for the expansion of services to treat a larger
population. Others maintained the belief that only by training an indigenous medical profession would they be effective
in alleviating suffering and disease on a broad scale. The missionary vision was to rejuvenate the Chinese nation through
the inculcation of Western science and Christian values.
Omar Kilborn's appeal in 1910 summarizes this vision: 'To
have a part in the uplift and in the moulding of what has
been in the past and is destined to be again, one of the
greatest nations of the earth!'[7] An evaluation of the missionary effort from a vantage point of eighty years later would
conclude that they were unsuccessful in achieving their goal
to bring Sichuan into the modern era. The complexities of
Chinese political and social developments have dwarfed Christian missionary influence in China. However, the small
medical elite they trained and nurtured have contributed in
no small way to the development of an indigenous profession. In this sense, through the 'multiplication of themselves,' the missionaries influenced the outcome of China's
medical modernization.

What of the Chinese recipients of this education? The students who were encouraged to roll between two cultures, to
be part of a university where 'two cultures embrace,' found
themselves facing a predicament which I have called cultural fragmentation. Like the Chinese students who studied
abroad in the 1920s and 1930s, they experienced value conflicts in their professional lives. Such a student was
described as 'rootless, denationalized, and detribalized ...
alienated from the folkways and customs of his people,

made accustomed to social and scientific affluence, dis-oriented by preoccupation with techniques and concerns of little relevance to his own society, and progressively drawn apart from genuine service to his community and nation.'[8] Although the WCUU alumni do not fit every aspect of this description, they had to overcome many dissonant exper-iences. The recognition of the social consequences of cross-cultural technology transfer has led to a recognition of the limitations of this process.[9]

At the same time, we must acknowledge that despite the obstacles, cultural diffusion did occur. Thomas Metzger, in his study of the predicament of neo-Confucian intellectuals in China, refers to the key part played by the reactions of those presented with foreign ideas. Metzger argues that in some cases, Chinese and Western values were congruous, and that therefore Western notions were acceptable to the Chinese intelligentsia. He discusses three aspects of Western assump-tions about modernization and points out their counterparts in Chinese thought. The first relates to the similarity of the Western belief in 'rapid cultural conversion' and the Chinese notion of 'sudden enlightenment.' The second is a compatibil-ity of the Christian and Buddhist notions of compassion and service. The third, and perhaps the most cogent for this dis-cussion, is the attitude towards technology. The foreigners were not alone in their zeal to harness nature in the service of material progress. There is an ancient tradition in China that reveres technical achievement.[10] One of the great legend-ary figures of Sichuan Province was Li Bing, a Qin dynasty engineer who harnessed the Min River and rechannelled it to irrigate the fertile Chengdu Plain. In honour of their achieve-ments, he and his son have been deified in two Daoist temples, with larger-than-life statues; and the story of the Guangxian irrigation system is well known in Sichuan. Chi-na's response to Western technology was to see it not so much as a threat to the status quo, but as a tool in China's material transformation. The threat was the destabilizing influence of the values that accompanied the knowledge and technology.

A Generation of Chinese Intellectuals

The socialization of the alumni of WCUU, the attitudes, beliefs, and values that they learned from their childhood experiences, their education, the political history of their times, and their careers, characterize them as a unique generation.[11] It is perhaps these characteristics that are most salient in our understanding of their role in modern China.

Unlike the literary elite – the writers and philosophers, and even the economists of contemporary China – this cohort did not commit their ideas to writing. As they were practitioners of an applied science, their only written publications would be scientific articles. Their values, beliefs, and attitudes have to be discerned from what they are willing to say about themselves, from an analysis of their personal histories, and from comparative studies of similar groups within the Chinese intelligentsia.

There have been some excellent studies of China's intellectual elites that are relevant to the study of this group's generational attributes.[12] The alumni themselves conceptualize their peers in terms of generation: the 1920s, 1930s, and 1940s graduates. Li Zehou and Vera Schwarcz present a typology of six generations of Chinese intellectuals.[13] Using Lu Xun's conceptualization of China's intellectual reformers from 1898 to the anti-Japanese War, Li and Schwarcz identified six groups that span the period 1898 to 1974.[14] Using the theoretical work of Karl Mannheim and Julian Marias, they identified 'key transforming historical events' that define the boundaries between generations.[15] Each of these generations is defined by its style, character, socialization, and spirit. For our purposes, the earlier groups coincide with the parents and grandparents of our cohort, the Anti-Japanese War group with the alumni, and the subsequent groups with their students.

The grandparents of this cohort were born into a conservative, patriarchal Confucian society. They believed in the traditional values of the scholar-official. They were moved by a certain patriotism, and in the quest for national salvation, many looked to foreign ideas, particularly Christianity and Western science, to see what could be learned and put to China's use. The parents of our alumni came to maturity around the time of the Revolution of 1911 and the May Fourth Movement of 1919. They experienced a radical shift in traditional social values and in the route to upward mobility, and encouraged their children to acquire modern technical and language skills to guarantee their livelihood in a rapidly changing society.

The alumni themselves were encouraged to seek autonomy from the chaos of unstable political times by mastering Western medical science. This would afford them professional status and the ability to cope with a changing environment. Although they were urban-centred and rather distant from the rural social revolution which was brewing from 1920 to 1949, they were galvanized by the Anti-Japanese War to work for their country. Their Chinese teachers, who had been raised during the May Fourth period, were more cosmopolitan than previous generations of intellectuals. They were aware of developments in the West and more receptive to foreign ideas. In conjunction with foreign professors, they passed on ideas of internationalism to their students.

Vera Schwarcz suggests that the national salvation movements of the 1930s and 1940s 'consumed the energies of their youth.'[16] They had less opportunity to study abroad than the May Fourth generation; many returned after the war to contribute to China's self-strengthening. After 1950, many wholeheartedly contributed to the Communist efforts to transform China, even though they were not committed Communists themselves. Described as 'patriotic idealists,'[17] they were perhaps the most disillusioned of the intellectuals. They were the targets of countless campaigns to reform bourgeois intellectuals, some more severe than others. It is a tribute to their strength of spirit that they returned phoenix-like after 1978 to become influential senior advisers in the rebuilding of the nation's medical education and research system.

The Role of a Modernizing Medical Elite

Although China's policy towards intellectuals shifted in 1978 towards the recognition of their role in modernization, there remains deeply entrenched resistance to intellectual influence. Sought as advisers to political reformers, they are perceived as a threat to many veteran cadres who continue to be obsessed with class struggle. Senior scientists perceive that it is difficult to convince the *lao ganbu*, the old cadres, of the important role of knowledge and expertise in production. This resistance is exacerbated by the traditional role of intellectuals as critics of the political system. While this role was ruthlessly suppressed by the Communists, the relaxation of social policy after 1978 led to the emergence of threats to the regime's political legitimacy. Intellectuals who were formerly isolated from each other began to form networks, and a circle around the renowned scientist Fang Li-zhi challenged the Communist system from within. Except for a minuscule number of 'establishment intellectuals,'[18] China's intellectual elites are not political elites. They have little access to political power, and they are further restrained by the absence of professional coalitions. After 1956, alumni associations were outlawed, and even informal gatherings were perceived as a threat to the state. Isolated in specialized schools and research institutes, with no mobility between institutions, intellectuals were atomized, with no professional autonomy or peer support. Only with the Open-Door policy in 1978 were they allowed to form associations, and these were for the purpose of seeking financial support from overseas alumni. When professional associations took on political agendas in 1989, they were again vigorously suppressed.[19] An analysis of the role of China's intellectuals in the state observes that 'civil society' is 'the dominant background of intellectual life in mainland China.'[20] In the development of science and technology, the state continues to play an interventionist role, constraining the autonomous and energetic development of a scientific elite. As Apter predicted,[21] and Richard Suttmeier notes in his analysis of the 'science-technology-politics' relationship,[22]

China's professional elites are more likely to be in conflict with political elites, as the latter struggle to maintain control of scientific expertise. The shifting models in education and research, between political correctness and research expertise (the 'red versus expert' conundrum) has further weakened the development of a scientific elite by interfering with the momentum and cumulative nature of scientific development.

The Limits of Cross-cultural Technology Transfer

Although medical knowledge and skills were undoubtedly imparted to the Chinese students of WCUU, there were a number of factors that confounded the unimpeded transfer of technology and ideas. The alumni were clearly receptive to Western education, however their response was tempered by their strong identification with Chinese culture. Exposed to Christianity and liberal-democratic values, they nonetheless did not convert to Christianity in significant numbers, and most avoided political involvement unless it was thrust upon them. In terms of being 'Westernized,' they were sincerely interested and attracted to Western ideas and culture, but rejected the notion of 'wholesale Westernization.' The professors most respected by the Chinese students were those who, like Leslie Kilborn, understood Chinese culture and had a command of the Chinese language and a deep respect for students and colleagues. When it came to choosing sides, however, the Chinese alumni, distasteful as Marxism may have been to them philosophically, had to choose the Chinese Communists, who seemed to offer the greatest hope for China's salvation in 1950.

The forced acceptance by WCUU alumni of the Communist repudiation of the Western model of medical education and care, however, was of minor significance compared with the disruption of their careers. The role of this medical elite in the development of a modern health-care system was profoundly limited by the state's dogmatic adherence to a series of shifting educational models. The cumulative and developmental nature of research, science curricula, pedagogy, and

institutional growth was severely hampered by the fluctu-
ations in China's science and educational policy. The maltreatment of Western-educated elites was further influenced
by Chinese foreign policy, which set up the West as the arch-
enemy of Communist China, and identified those associated
with the West as 'lackeys,' witting or unwitting, of American
imperialism. This castigation of the Western-educated alumni
restricted their ability to contribute in their full capacity to
China's medical modernization. On the one hand, the state
relied on them for their expertise; on the other, it distrusted
them as petty bourgeois intellectuals.

What is the significance of this cross-cultural encounter in
technology transfer? The story of the interaction of Western
medical missionaries, and Chinese students, and of the development over time of the careers of a Western-educated elite
in China, makes us acutely aware of the range of factors that
influence technology transfer through the transfer of knowledge. In retrospect, one could have anticipated various out-
comes of this transfer, moderated by the political climate of
post-revolutionary China. Taking the approach of this study,
one could assess the application of contemporary foreign
assistance programs in technology transfer in China and else-
where. What kind of knowledge and technologies could survive the onslaught experienced by our cohort of medical
elites?

It is a phenomenon of this process of technology transfer
that the alumni maintained their faith in the elitist model
introduced by the missionaries and the first generation of
Western-educated Chinese professors. The physician-scientist,
motivated by the spirit of service and excellence, is the standard for the top echelon of physicians in China. This standard
has been challenged by the continuing demand to provide
health care to a population that exceeds one billion people.
Moreover, the most highly trained medical elite in the country are lured abroad by Western research funds and the opportunity to work in the most sophisticated medical centres in
the world. The 1980s and 1990s generation of medical scientists who go abroad have for the most part been unwilling to

return to China to bear the frustrations endured by their teachers, the *laoyibei zhishifenzi* (literally, the old generation intellectuals), the backbone of the intellectual elite. The old alumni, frustrated at every turn by shifting policies and an entrenched political authority that was unsympathetic to their ideas, nonetheless maintained the hope that the modern medicine that they transported across the threshold of 1949 would continue to develop in China. Like a flame flickering in the wind, they have struggled to keep the spirit of international scientific and professional excellence alive in themselves and, most important, in their students. This legacy, passed on from the Western medical missionaries to their Chinese students, is the essence of the collaboration between China and the West during the first half of the twentieth century.

Appendix:
Questionnaire for Alumni of West China Union University College of Medicine and Dentistry

Instructions: Please answer these questions as fully as possible. If there is a question which you cannot answer, please go on to the next question. You may answer in either Chinese or English. [The questionnaire was in both languages; only the English is reprinted here.]

Name (pinyin)   Chinese characters

University degree

Year of graduation

Occupation

I Background

1. Year of birth

2. Place of birth

3. Family

   a) What was your father's occupation?

   b) What was your mother's occupation?

   c) What was your family's religious background?

   d) Siblings (please complete information for each sibling.)

   Male/female   Level of education   Occupation

e) Children

Male/female   *Level of education*   *Occupation*

f) Spouse: Name
   Level of education
   Occupation
   If university graduate, which university?

4. Early Education (please check the appropriate box.)

Type of School	Government	Missionary	*Foreign secular*
Primary	☐	☐	☐
Lower middle school	☐	☐	☐
Upper middle school	☐	☐	☐
Comments			

II Student life – undergraduate

1. What dates did you attend university?

2. Why did you choose to attend West China Union University?

3. Who provided support while you were at university?

4. Why did you choose medicine/dentistry/pharmacy?

5. What is your subspecialty and how did you choose it?
6. Who were the most influential professors and why?
7. Perceptions of HuaDa
   a) What was WCUU's reputation? compared to PUMC,
      National Central, and other medical schools in China?
   b) What were the educational goals of professors?
   c) What were the goals of the university?

8. Are there any courses which you wish to comment on?

9. Describe faculty/student relations.

10. a) Were you aware of faculty political sympathies?
    b) Did any faculty members try to influence your political
       beliefs?

11. Students
    a) How many started in your class? How many graduates?
    b) What extracurricular activities did you participate in?

(Please check the appropriate boxes.)
☐ choir
☐ sports
☐ political groups
☐ Bible study
☐ other _____
Please comment on the above.

   c) Did students socialize with each other based on:
☐ geographic origin
☐ socioeconomic background
☐ generations (1930s, 1940s)
☐ faculty of studies

12. Clinical training
   a) In which hospital did you do your clinical training?
   b) Did you ever work at a station hospital (e.g., Zegong, Leshan, etc.)?
   c) Did the interns belong to a union or organization?
   d) What were the working conditions during your training?
      i.   working hours
      ii. patient load
      iii. working relations with staff doctors
   e) Did you treat foreign patients?
   f) How did Chinese patients respond to being treated by a foreign-trained doctor?
   g) What was your position in society compared to that of a traditional Chinese doctor?

13. Can you comment on the devolution of responsibility and authority from foreign professors to Chinese professors?

III Career after HuaDa

1. Did you do postgraduate study?
   a) Where?
   b) What subject?

2. Describe your career during the 1950s.

3. Were you criticized during the 1957 Anti-Rightist Movement? Were you labelled a 'Rightist'?

4. Describe your career during the 1960s.

5. What were your experiences during the Cultural Revolution? *If you wish to use these questions as a guideline, they may be helpful in answering question 5.*

    1. *Were you part of a revolutionary rebel organization during the Cultural Revolution?*

    2. *Were you subjected to mass criticism? What were you labelled as?*

    3. *Were you detained and subjected to political investigation? For how long and for what issues?*

    4. *Was your home ever searched by Red Guards or other radicals?*

    5. *Were your professional books and journals confiscated or destroyed?*

    6. *Were you allowed to continue your professional work?*

    7. *Did your children suffer because of your problems?*

    8. *Were you sent to a May 7 Cadre School? Where was the school? How long were you there?*

    9. *When were you released from school? Did you return to work in your unit? Were you incorporated into a '3-in-1 leading group' of a revolutionary committee?*

    10. *How severe were the struggles in your work unit? How did your treatment compare with that of your colleagues?*

    11. *Any additional comments?*

6. What has your position been since 1978?

7. Do you have any party affiliation?

8. Do you have any religious affiliation?

IV Ideas about medical development (Please be as specific as you can.)

1. How would you define 'modern medicine'?

2. What is your perception of present med/dent/pharm education at HuaDa?
   a) advantages:
   b) problems:

3. What proposals do you have for the development of medical education in China/HuaDa in future?

Request for confidentiality

I,_____, request that my name not be used in any publication. I understand that the information in this questionnaire will be used as part of a study of West China Union University's College of Medicine and Dentistry.

_____

Signature

_____

Date

Illustration Credits

Archives of the United Church of Canada, Victoria University, University of Toronto: Methodist missionaries in Sichuan; staff of the Chengdu hospital; first Canadian medical missionaries; opening of the Si Sheng Ci Men's Hospital; baby welfare clinic; Dr F. Allan with patients; Drs Kilborn in the operating room; E.N. Meuser; early graduating class in medicine; women, class of 1937; medical faculty of the WCUU; Dr L. Dsang and family; staff of the Women's Hospital; dentistry professors, graduates, and students; Dr L. Kilborn with students; Dr W.R. Morse's anatomy class; first building used as a medical college; Dr Morse instructing students; Dr C. Best instructing students; Dr J.E. Thompson with student; Dr Luo Guang-bi and Dr Best; Dr J. Beech; Si Sheng Ci Men's Hospital; Ziliujing hospital; teaching hospital; Dr Morse in biology building; Map 1

Our West China Mission (Toronto: The Missionary Society of the Methodist Church, 1920): Map 2

Dr H. Schipper: president's residence; lotus pond; Dr H. Yoh

frontispiece: calligraphy by Liu Guo-wu, Chengdu, Sichuan

Notes

Introduction

1 These included the Methodist Church of Canada, Church Missionary Society of England, American Baptist Foreign Mission Society, Friends Service Council of England, and Methodist Episcopal Church of the United States.
2 For an excellent discussion of this process and the historical background to the instrumentalization of higher education in China, see Ruth Hayhoe, *China's Universities and the Open Door* (Armonk, NY: M.E. Sharpe 1989).
3 Michael F. Seefeldt, 'Cultural Considerations for Evaluation Consulting in the Egyptian Context,' in M.Q. Patton, ed., *Cultural Evaluation, New Directions for Program Evaluation*, no. 25 (1985), 75
4 M.L. Smith and C.V. Glass, *Research and Evaluation in Education and the Social Sciences* (Englewood Cliffs, NJ: Prentice-Hall 1987)
5 *Huaxi Yike Daxue Jin Xi*, 1910–1985 (West China University of Medical Sciences, Present and Past; Chengdu: West China University of Medical Sciences school history publication committee 1985). Dr Lewis Walmsley has written an excellent short history, *West China Union University* (New York: United Board for Christian Higher Education in Asia 1974).
6 See chapter 5, 'Students in China's Christian Colleges.'
7 These included several heart-rending letters from Austrian and German Jewish doctors requesting asylum in West China before the escalation of Hitler's extermination campaign. Although there were several European Jewish refugees among the students and

faculty in the 1940s, it is not known whether any of these letters received a positive response.

8 Studies using the generational approach to Chinese intellectuals include: Sally Borthwick, *Education and Social Change in China: The Beginning of the Modern Era* (Stanford: Hoover Institution Press 1983); Yue Daiyun and Carolyn Wakeman, *To The Storm: The Odyssey of a Revolutionary Chinese Woman* (Berkeley: University of California Press 1985); Li Zehou and Vera Schwarcz, 'Six Generations of Modern Chinese Intellectuals,' *Chinese Studies in History* 17(2): 42–56 (Winter 1983–4); Vera Schwarcz, 'Behind a Partially-Open Door: Chinese Intellectuals and the Post-Mao Reform Process,' *Pacific Affairs* 59(4): 577–604 (1986); John Israel, *Student Nationalism in China, 1927–1937* (Stanford: Stanford University Press 1966); Anne F. Thurston, *Enemies of the People: The Ordeal of the Intellectuals in China's Great Cultural Revolution* (Cambridge, Mass.: Harvard University Press 1988); Vera Schwarcz, 'Afterword,' and John Israel, 'Foreword,' in T. Cheek and C. Hamrin, *China's Establishment Intellectuals* (Armonk, NY: M.E. Sharpe 1986). A review of Western scholarly literature on 'generations' as an approach to understanding historical change can be found in Julian Marias, *Generations: A Historical Method*, trans. Harold C. Raley (Alabama: University of Alabama Press 1979).

9 A year after the initial visit to Chengdu, the author received a list of names and addresses of 131 alumni. This list, augmented by contact made from interviews with alumni already identified, formed the basis for the questionnaire distribution. In May 1989 (a year after the questionnaires had been distributed, returned, translated, and analysed), it was discovered that the list had been preselected from a more complete list, not at the author's disposal. The alumni had apparently been selected according to who was 'most likely to respond.' The drastic change in China's political climate in June 1989, the advancing age of this cohort, and the practical constraints of research led to the decision to accept this sample as the only available group for study.

10 The author is grateful to Professor Beth Goldstein of the University of Kentucky (Lexington) for her expert assistance in developing the questionnaire and for her suggestions on the details of distribution to ensure maximum return.

11 These include Chengdu, Beijing, Tianjin, Shanghai, Leshan (Sichuan), and Hong Kong.

Chapter 1

1 See Arthur Waley, *The Opium War through Chinese Eyes* (London: George Allen and Unwin 1958).

2 Mary C. Wright, ed., *The Last Stand of Chinese Conservatism: The T'ung-chih Restoration, 1862–1874* (Stanford: Stanford University Press 1957), 239–40, passim

3 Li Chien-nung, *The Political History of China, 1840–1928* (Stanford: Stanford University Press 1956), 91–2, passim

4 The Chinese phrase is 'Zhong wei ti; Xi wei yong.' Wright, *Last Stand*, 1 and D.W. Treadgold, *The West in Russia and China*, vol. 2, China, 1852–1949 (Cambridge: Cambridge University Press 1973), 101–2

5 See C.H. Peake, 'Some Aspects of the Introduction of Modern Science into China,' *Isis*, 22(63): 173–219 (December 1934).

6 Jonathan Spence, *To Change China: Western Advisers in China, 1620–1960* (New York: Penguin 1980)

7 J.C. Thomson, Jr, *While China Faced West; American Reformers in Nationalist China, 1928–1937* (Cambridge, Mass.: Harvard University Press 1969), 235

8 See Thomson, ibid.: P.R. Bohr, *Famine in China and the Missionary: Timothy Richard as a Relief Administrator and Advocate of National Reform, 1876–1884* (Cambridge, Mass.: Harvard East Asian Monograph 1972); and W.H. Mallory, *China, Land of Famine* (New York 1926).

9 John King Fairbank, *The United States and China* (New York: Viking Press 1962), 142; and editor, *The Missionary Enterprise in China and America* (Cambridge, Mass.: Harvard University Press 1974, 'Introduction,' 1, passim

10 Fairbank, *The Missionary Enterprise*, 10

11 C.H. Peake, 'Some Aspects,' 173

12 Harold D. Lasswell, 'Commentary,' *Far Eastern Quarterly* 12(2): 170 (Feb. 1953)

13 Ralph Croizier, *Traditional Medicine in Modern China: Science, Nationalism, and the Tensions of Cultural Change* (Cambridge, Mass.: Harvard University Press 1968), 36

14 Peter Buck, *American Science and Modern China, 1876–1936* (Cambridge: Cambridge University Press 1980), chap. 2, 9, 39, 44

15 For example: John Z. Bowers, MD *Western Medicine in a Chinese Palace: Peking Medical College, 1917–1951* (New York: Josiah Macy, Jr., Foundation 1972); John Z. Bowers, and Elizabeth F.

Purcell, eds. *Medicine and Society in China* (New York: Josiah Macy, Jr., Foundation 1974); Mary Brown Bullock, 'The Rockefeller Foundation in China: Philanthropy, Peking Union Medical College, and Public Health' (Ph.D. dissertation, Stanford University 1973); Nigel Cameron. *Barbarians and Mandarins* (Chicago: University of Chicago Press 1970); R. Holden, *Yale in China: The Mainland 1901–1951* (New Haven, Conn.: Yale in China Association, 1964); I.T. Hyatt, Jr., 'Protestant Missions in China, 1877–1890: The Institutionalization of Good Works,' in Liu Kwang-ching, ed., *American Missionaries in China* (Cambridge, Mass.: Harvard East Asian Monograph 1966), 93–128; A. Kleinman et al., *Medicine in Chinese Cultures: Comparative Studies of Health Care in Chinese and Other Societies* (DHEW(NIH) 1975), 75–653, especially Ralph Croizier, 'Medicine and Modernization in China,' 21–35; AnElissa Lucas, 'Chinese Medical "Modernization" in Comparative Historical Perspective' (Ph.D. dissertation, Harvard University 1977); J.G. Lutz, *China and the Christian Colleges, 1850–1950* (Ithaca: Cornell University Press 1971); Carl F. Nathan, *Plague Prevention and Politics in Manchuria 1910–1931* (Cambridge, Mass.: Harvard University Press 1967); Joseph Needham, *Within the Four Seas: The Dialogue of East and West* (London: George Allen and Unwin 1969); Clara A. Nutting, 'Health Department,' in *The Healthy Village, An Experiment in Visual Education in West China* (UNESCO 1951); W. Reeves, Jr., 'Sino-American Cooperation in Medicine: The Origins of Hsiang-Ya (1902–1914),' in Liu ed., *American Missionaries*, 129–82; J. Spence, *To Change China* (Harmondsworth: Penguin 1980); James C. Thomson, Jr., *While China Faced West* (Cambridge, Mass.: Harvard University Press 1969); Philip West, *Yenching University and Sino-Western Relations, 1916–1952* (Cambridge, Mass.: Harvard University Press 1976); K. Chimin Wong, and Wu Lien Teh, *History of Chinese Medicine* (Shanghai: National Quarantine Service 1936), 2nd ed. revised.

16 A.A. Koskinen, *Missionary Influence as a Political Factor in the Pacific Islands* (Helsinki: 1953)

17 R.I. Rotberg, *Christian Missionaries in the Creation of Northern Rhodesia, 1880–1924* (Princeton, NJ: Princeton University Press 1965)

18 Among these studies are: J.F. Ade Ayaji, *Christian Missions in Nigeria, 1841–1891: The Making of a New Elite* (Evanston: Northwestern University Press, 1965); E.A. Ayandele, *The*

Missionary Impact on Modern Nigeria, 1842–1914 (New York: Humanities Press 1967); M.D. Markowitz, *Cross and Sword: The Political Role of Christian Missions in the Belgian Congo, 1908–1960* (Stanford: Hoover Institution Press, 1973); J. McCracken, *Politics and Christianity in Malawi 1975–1940* (Cambridge: Cambrdige University Press, 1977); K.N. Mufuka, *Missions and Politics in Malawi* (Kingston, Ont.: Limestone Press 1977); R. Oliver, *The Missionary Factor in East Africa* (London: Longman, 1952); A. Schweitzer, *On the Edge of the Primeval Forest* (London: Adam and Charles Black 1948). Examples from the Indian subcontinent include K.M. De Silva, *Social Policy and Missionary Organizations in Ceylon, 1840–1855* (London: Longmans 1965), and E.D. Potts, *British Baptist Missionaries in India, 1793–1837* (Cambridge: Cambridge University Press 1967).

19 The examples of the latter include Denis Goulet, *The Uncertain Promise: Value Conflicts in Technology Transfer* (New York: IDOC 1977 and J. Ramesh, and C. Weiss, eds., *Mobilizing Technology for World Development* (New York: Praeger 1979).

20 Ralph Braibanti, 'Political Development: Contextual nonlinear perspectives', *Politikon* 3(2): 6–18 (October 1976). See also R. Braibanti and J. Spengler, *Tradition, Values, and Socio-Economic Development* (Durham, NC: Duke University 1961), particularly the following chapters: M.J. Herskovits, 'Economic Change and Cultural Dynamics,' 114–38; Braibanti, 'Relevance of Political Science to the Study of Underdeveloped Areas,' 139–80, and J.D. Montgomery, 'Political Dimensions of Foreign Aid,' 243–75. See also D.M. Apter, *The Politics of Modernization* (Chicago: University of Chicago Press 1965), 174.

21 See two detailed reports by Arthur Waldron of Princeton University on the progression of this trend and on the cooperation with a group of American and Canadian researchers organized by Waldron and funded by the Luce Foundation through the History of Christianity in China project of the University of Kansas. Arthur Waldron, 'Possibilities for Cooperative Archival Research on the History of Christian Higher Education in China: Report of an Exploratory Visit to the People's Republic of China June 1986.' (unpublished report, Princeton University, July 1989); and Arthur Waldron, 'Report on the First International Conference on the Study of Christian Colleges in China, held at Huazhong Normal University, June 1–3, 1989.' (unpublished report, Princeton University, July 1989)

22 Although Canada did not have a history of military involvement in China, it was closely identified with 'America.' Had the Canadian government accepted a recommendation to appoint Leslie Kilborn, the Dean of Medicine at West China Union University, as ambassador to Chongqing during the anti-Japanese war, the Communists would have been able to argue even more forcefully that *Hua Da* was a tool of Western imperialism.

23 Mao Zedong, *Selected Works*, (Beijing: People's Publishing House 1960), vol. 4, 438

24 Ibid., 437

25 Waldron, 'Possibilities for Cooperative Archival Research'; see also Waldron's 'Report on the First international Conference.'

26 These studies include He Di, 'Yenjing University and Educational Modernization in China', (Beijing: Institute of American Studies, Chinese Academy of Social Sciences, 1989); Shi Jinghuan, 'Studies in Educational Thoughts and Activities of C.W. Mateer and J.L. Stuart,' Ph.D. thesis, Beijing Normal University 1989).

27 Michel Bonnin and Yves Chevrier, 'The Intellectual and the State: Social Dynamics of Intellectual Autonomy during the Post-Mao Era,' *China Quarterly*, 127: 572 (Sept. 1991)

28 Listed in Vera Schwarcz, 'Afterword,' in Cheek and Hamrin, *China's Establishment Intellectuals* (Armonk, NY: M.E. Sharpe 1986), 248

29 See Richard Suttmeier's discussion of the relationship between science, technology, and politics, in 'Science, Technology, and China's Political Future – A Framework for Analysis,' in Denis Simon and Merle Goldman, eds., *Science and Technology in Post-Mao China* (Cambridge, Mass.: Harvard University Press 1989), 375–96.

30 David Apter, *The Politics of Modernization* (Chicago: University of Chicago Press 1965), 124, 175, 176

31 Bonnin and Chevrier, 'The Intellectual and the State,' 572

32 Gordon White, *Party and Professionals: The Political Role of Teachers in Contemporary China* (Armonk, NY: M.E. Sharpe 1981), 91, 90

33 Denis Simon, 'China's Scientists and Technologists in the Post-Mao Era: A Retrospective and Prospective Glimpse,' in Goldman, Cheek, and Hamrin, *China's Intellectuals and the State* (N.Y.: M.E. Sharpe 1987), 144

34 L.A. Schneider, 'Learning from Russia: Lysenkoism and the Fate of

Genetics in China, 1950–1986, 'in Simon and Goldman, *Science and Technology*, 45–65

35 Sally Borthwick, *Education and Social Change in China* (Stanford: Hoover Institution Press 1983), p. 140, 153

36 Merle Goldman and Denis Simon, 'The Onset of China's New Technological Revolution,' in Simon and Goldman, *Science and Technology*, 3, 6.

37 Denis Simon, citing Leo Orleans, in 'China's Scientists,' in Goldman et al., *China's Intellectuals*, 131

38 White, *Party and Professionals*, 11–12, 67

39 Goldman and Simon, *Science and Technology*, 13

40 Li Honglin, 'Socialism and Opening to the Outside World,' *People's Daily* (15 Oct. 1984), 5, cited in Goldman and Simon, *Science and Technology* 14

41 Bonnin and Chevrier, 'The Intellectual and the State.' 569–70

42 Simon, 'China's Scientists and Technologists,' 144–5

43 Vera Schwarcz, in Cheek and Hamrin, *China's Establishment*, 248, 249

44 William Kirby, 'Technocratic Organization and Technological Development in China: The Nationalist Experience and Legacy, 1928–1953,' in Simon and Goldman, *Science and Technology*, 43

45 Apter, *Politics*, 132, 133

Chapter 2

1 E.I. Hart, *Virgil C. Hart: Missionary Statesman (Founder of the American and Canadian Missions in Central and West China)* (Toronto: McClelland, Goodchild, and Stewart 1917) 222, 223

2 United Church of Canada Archives (UCA), West China Union University (WCUU) pamphlet, 'Spend Ten Minutes in China,' 1919–20?

3 UCA-West China Mission (WCM) pamphlet, 'A Statement of Mission Plant' (Toronto: Methodist Mission Rooms 1910)

4 UCA, WCUU, 'Spend Ten Minutes'

5 The Methodist Church amalgamated in 1925 with two other Protestant denominations to form the United Church of Canada.

6 V.C Hart, *Western China* (Boston: Tickner 1888), 281. See also E.R. Huc's description in 1855 in *The Chinese Empire*, quoted in Hsiao Kung-chuan, *Rural China: Imperial Control in the Nineteenth Century* (Seattle: University of Washington Press 1960), 13.

7 G.W. Skinner, 'Marketing and Social Structure in Rural China, Part II,' *Journal of Asian Studies* 24(2): 204, 225–7

8 UCA-WCM pamphlet, 'A Statement,' 8

9 M.T. Stauffer, ed., *The Christian Occupation of China* (Shanghai: China Continuation Committee 1922) Appendix B, iii

10 The names of the stations are given in *pinyin* spelling. The missionaries did not use standard or consistent spellings for place names or personal names.

11 *Our West China Mission* (Toronto: Missionary Society of the Methodist Church 1920), 103

12 UCC-MCC-GBM-WCM 1–4, 'The Place of Medical Missions in Missionary Work.' This is a Methodist Church of Canada document, pre-dating 1925.

13 *Our West China Mission*, 103–4, 230

14 Department of External Affairs Archives (DEA) 4558-40C, Victor Odlum to H.L. Keenleyside, 16 June 1943

15 Personal correspondence, E.R. Cunningham to family, 26 June 1925

16 See R.P. Hommel, *China at Work* (New York: John Day 1937; Cambridge, Mass.: MIT Press 1969, 114–17); and A. Feuerwerker, *The Chinese Economy, 1912–1949* (University of Michigan: Michigan Papers in Chinese Studies, no. 1, 1968), 49–50.

17 See John Fairbank and Teng Ssu-yu, eds. *China's Response to the West: A Documentary Survey, 1839–1923* (Cambridge, Mass.: Harvard University Press 1954; New York: Atheneum 1973, 112).

18 UCA, 'Station and Institutional Reports,' 1925, 16.

19 Interview with Mrs Ralph Hayward, 22 Feb. 1978, Toronto, Canada. Mrs Hayward was the wife of a medical missionary stationed at Jiading.

20 A. Hosie, *Three Years in Western China* (London: George Philip 1890), chap. 11

21 For details of these events, see John Munro, *Beyond the Moon Gate* (adapted from the diaries of Margaret Outerbridge; Vancouver: Douglas and McIntyre 1990). Also Karen Minden, 'Missionaries, Medicine, and Modernization: Canadian Missionaries in Sichuan, 1925–1952' (Ph.D. dissertation, York University, Toronto 1981).

22 *Our West China Mission*, 184

23 Ibid., 123

24 Ibid., 101–2

25 Robert Kapp, *Szechwan and the Chinese Republic* (New Haven, Conn., and London: Yale University Press (1973), and *The Story of*

the *Missions of the United Church of Canada in China* (Toronto: Ryerson Press, 1928), 114

26 United Church of Canada, Board of Foreign Missions, *Forward with China*, (Toronto: Committee on Literature, General Publicity and Missionary Education 1928), 222

27 *Our West China Mission*, 109.

28 Ibid., 110.

29 UCC-BFM-WCM 1-1, June 1926

30 'On Being Removed from Hsien-yang and Sent to Chung-chou,' 818 AD This poem was given to the author from the file of a medical missionary. It may be attributable to Bai Juyi, a Tang poet who was appointed governor of Zhongzhou in 818 AD. Several biographical references report that he was very lonely at this post. (My thanks to an anonymous reviewer for suggesting Bai Juyi as the likely author.)

31 Detailed descriptions and analysis can be found in Minden, 'Missionaries, Medicine and Modernization,' chap. 5 and 6.

32 Hart, *Western China*, 296

33 O.R. Joliffe, 'The Field,' in *Our West China Mission*, 101–2

34 *Our West China Mission*, 102; and Kapp, *Szechwan*, 34

35 A. Doak Barnett, *China on the Eve of Communist Takeover* (New York: Praeger 1963), 143

36 Kapp, *Szechwan*, 110-11

37 The traditional roles of the gentry, police, and magistrates are discussed in profound detail in Hsiao, *Rural China*. A brief political history of the province and a detailed description of the political organization of one county can be found in Barnett, *China on the Eve*, chap. 10. Missionary accounts include *Our West China Mission* and numerous archival references.

38 Geraldine Hartwell, 'Twelfth Letter Home,' Rongxian, July–Sept. 1945. UCA biographical files

39 Kapp, *Szechwan*, 29

40 Toller (Chunking) to Peiping, 22 Sept. 1930, FO 228/4208, Doss. 32s, cited in ibid., 58

41 Hsiao, *Rural China*, 269–70. See also Etienne Balazs, *Chinese Civilization and Bureaucracy* (New Haven, Conn., and London: Yale University Press 1964); Chang Chung-li, *The Chinese Gentry* (Seattle: University of Washington Press 1955); and Fei Hsiao-tung, *China's Gentry*, (Chicago: University of Chicago Press 1953).

42 Barnett, *China on the Eve*, 129

43 *Our West China Mission*, 54

Chapter 3

1 West China University of Medical Sciences (WCUMS) Archives, Yuan Shi-kai's inscription to Dr Joseph Beech, 1914; author's translation

2 United Church of Canada Archives (UCA) MCCNB-WCCU, box 6, file 87 (no date, but published before church union in 1925)

3 Nathan Sivin, 'Science in China's Past,' in Leo Orleans, ed., *Science in Contemporary China* (Stanford: Stanford University Press 1980), 26.

4 Marion Levy, Jr., *Modernization and the Structure of Societies* (Princeton: Princeton University Press 1966), 467

5 UCA, 1

6 W.J.R. Morse, 'Medical Education in a Mission School,' *Chinese Medical Journal* 49: 875 (1935)

7 Karen Minden, 'Missionaries, Medicine, and Modernization: Canadian Medical Missionaries in Sichuan, 1925–1952' (Ph.D. dissertation, York University, Toronto 1981), passim; Minden, 'The Multiplication of Ourselves: Canadian Medical Missionaries in West China,' in Ruth Hayhoe and Marianne Bastid, eds., *China's Education and the Industrialized World: Studies in Cultural Transfer* (Armonk, NY: M.E. Sharpe 1987), 139–57

8 The other denominations were the Church Missionary Society of England, American Baptist Foreign Mission Society, Friends Service Council of England, and Methodist Episcopal Church of the United States. (See letterhead, Board of Governors of the West China Union University, WCM-BFM-WCUU files.) The early history of the WCUU is detailed in *Our West China Mission* (Toronto: Missionary Society of the Methodist Church 1920), 358–70. A complete history of the university can be found in Lewis Walmsley, *West China Union University* (New York: United Board for Christian Higher Education in Asia 1974). Walmsley was a missionary in West China and head of the Canadian School for children of missionaries.

9 UCC-BFM-WCUU 12–18, Board of Governors of the West China Union University

10 Ibid., 'Twenty-five years of Dentistry'

11 UCC-BFM-WCUU 12-295, Institute of Biochemistry at the West China Union University, 1948

12 UCA biographical files, 'E.N. Meuser.'

13 UCC-BFM-WCM 12-312, E.N. Meuser to Gallagher, 20 Jan. 1949

14　UCC-BFM-WCM 12-295, J.H. Arnup to L.G. Kilborn, 10 Feb. 1948

15　UCC-BFM-WCM 5-107, 'Report of Work by E.N. Meuser,' 1934

16　UCA-WCUU pamphlet, 'The West China Union University, 1910-1939.'

17　M. Bliss, *A Canadian Millionaire: The Life and Business Times of Sir Joseph Flavelle Bart, 1858–1939* (Toronto: Macmillan 1978), 496–7

18　RAC IIV 2B9-158-1154, 'Replies to Questionnaire from Dr Claude E. Forkner, Director, China Medical Board,' 1943

19　Chow Tse-tsung, *The May Fourth Movement: Intellectual Revolution in Modern China* (Stanford: Stanford University Press 1960), 327–30

20　The Chinese version and English translation of the school song were provided by Professor Sung Ruyao in Beijing. The translation was revised with the assistance of Song Xiaoping and Terry Russell, my colleagues at the University of Manitoba.

21　WCUMS Archives, *Sili Huaxi Xiehe Daxue Yilan*, in School Catalogue, 1941, 5

22　O.L. Kilborn, *Heal The Sick: An Appeal for Medical Missions in China* (Toronto: Missionary Society of the Methodist Church 1910), 220

23　UCC-BFM-WCUU 12-18, College of Medicine and Dentistry, 1942

24　UCA-WCUU, 'Spend Ten Minutes,' 15

25　UCA (uncatalogued), 'Report of the Special Committee on Policy (Medical Work),' 1936, 8–9

26　UCA-WCUU, 'West China Union University,' 9

27　UCA-BFM-WCM 6-135, L.G. Kilborn to J.H. Arnup, 2 Aug. 1937, 3. See also *Our West China Mission*, 368, 'Our Contribution.'

28　UCA-WCUU, 'West China Union University,' 9

29　UCC-BFM-WCM 1-1, 'West China Union University Needs.' The total medical budget was $750,000 out of a total university budget of $1,000,000. This included the departments of medicine, physics, biology, and chemistry (which taught medical students), and the hospitals.

30　UCC-BFM-WCM 1-4, Williams to J. Endicott, 24 Feb. 1926

31　UCC-BFM-WCM 5-100, J. Endicott to Gerald Bell, 26 July 1934

32　UCA, 'Report of the Special Committee on Policy,' 8

33　O.L. Kilborn, *Heal the Sick*, 223

34　UCA-WCUU, 'Spend Ten Minutes'

35　*Our West China Mission*, 396

36　RAC IV2B7-158-1154 CMB, 'Twenty-five Years of Dentistry,' 1942.

(See also UCC-BFM-WCUU 12-18.)

37 UCC-BFM-WCM 5-107, '1934 Report of Work by E.N. Meuser'

38 UCC-BFM-WCM 2-12, 'Report by Wm. Band, Sino-British Science Cooperative Office of the British Council,' Chongqing, 1944

39 UCC-BFM-WCM 4-95, H.B. Collier, 'Annual Report of Work: 1933,' 2

40 UCA China pamphlet series 1-29, 'Mission Legislation,' Chengdu, 1916. In an interview, Dr J. Endicott mentioned that one of his Chinese colleagues claimed that there were no fewer than thirteen virgin births reported in Chinese history.

41 For example, see UCC-BFM-WCM 5-121, 'Report of Work for the Year 1935,' R.C. Spooner (Department of Chemistry), 2, and Ibid. 4-92, H.B. Collier to J. Endicott, 30 Aug. 1933, 3

42 This is discussed in detail in chapter 4 of this book.

43 G.W. Sarvis, *Laymen's Foreign Missions Inquiry, Factfinders' Reports: China* vol. 5, suppl. 2, (New York 1933), 601

44 This standard was adopted after the Flexner Report was published in 1910. (It has been referred to as 'The Hopkins Model' after Johns Hopkins Medical School in Baltimore). See chapter 4 of this book for a more detailed discussion.

45 RAC IV 2B9-158-1154, W.P. Fenn, General Secretary, 17 Sept. 1963

46 Ibid., 'Replies to Questionnaire from Dr Claude Forkner,' Director, China Medical Board, 1943

47 RAC IV2B9-158-1156, L.G. Kilborn to Gregg, 1 July 1946. Also see the University of Toronto Faculty of Medicine Calendars, 1933 to 1946, 1933–4, 39

48 UCC-BFM-WCM 4-83, 'Report of Work, 1932,' L.G. Kilborn. This may have been an attempt to adapt the Rockefeller Peking Union Medical College system of eight years of training. The PUMC goal was to train medical researchers who would staff university medical schools. It was not practical for WCUU to follow this model, which depended on generous funding and adequate staff.

49 RAV IV2B9-158-1154, 'West China Union University College of Medicine and Dentistry (1937–9),' 1

50 RAC RG 4-9-2109, Stevenson, May 1926

51 UCC-BFM-WCM 3-66, 'Report of Work of the United Church of Canada West China Mission,' 1931, 15

52 RAC IV2B9-158-1154, 'Answers by the Department of Pharmacy of the West China Union University,' 14 Aug. 1944, 5

53 O.L. Kilborn, *Heal the Sick*, 224

54 W.J.R. Morse, '*Medical Education*,' 873

55 Ibid., 870, 875

56 National Central University Medical College was housed on
   WCUU's campus from 1937–41. Its shorter curriculum made integration of students difficult. Qilu Medical School students and faculty
   arrived in 1937, and PUMC in 1941, with both staying until the end
   of the war in 1945. WCUU was the only medical school in unoccupied China.
57 Personal communication from Dr George Deng, one of the
   residents in the program.
58 Hu Ding-an, 'Speech to the Graduating Class of 1944,' *Huaxi Yixun*
   (West China Medical Bulletin) 1: 93–5 (June 1944)
59 President Fong Shuxuan, quoted in *Huaxi Xiaokan* (West China
   Bulletin), 14 May 1949, 94
60 Li Ting-An, 'Control of Contagion and the Medical System,' *Huaxi
   Yixun* 1: 153–7 (Dec. 1944)
61 DEA 7988-40C, Office of Strategic Services, R & A no. 951, 'China's
   Destiny,' 15 July 1943, 10. This document is an analysis of Chiang
   Kai-shek's book of the same title.
62 UCC-BFM-WCM, 'Station and Institutional Reports,' 1925, 69
63 Sarvis, *Laymen's Foreign Missions Inquiry*, 602–3
64 UCC-BFM-WCM 2-41, L.G. Kilborn to J. Endicott, 9 Feb. 1929, 3
65 UCC-BFM-WCM 3-51, 'Report of Work,' 1930, L.G. Kilborn, 1
66 UCC-BFM-WCM 4-73, Gerald Bell to J. Endicott, 15 June 1932, 2, 3
67 UCC-BFM-WCM 4-92, L.G. Kilborn to J. Endicott, 1 Feb. 1933, 2
68 Ibid., J. Endicott to L.G. Kilborn, 28 Apr. 1933
69 UCC-BFM-WCM 5-99, Gerald Bell to J. Endicott, 22 Feb. 1934, 26, and
   UCC-BFM-WCM 4-92, 'Teaching of Surgery,' E.C. Wilford, July 1933
70 Ibid., 6-122, Gerald Bell to J. Endicott, 9 June 1936, 3
71 Ibid., 5-107, 'Report of Work,' 1934, H.B. Collier
72 RAC RG 1 Ser. 601-21-195, S.N. Cheer (dean of National Central
   Faculty of Medicine, Chengdu) to R.S. Greene (Rockefeller
   Foundation, China Medical Board), 16 Jan. 1939, 4
73 UCC-BFM-WCMU 3-12, 'News Notes,' no. 2, 1937, 7
74 W.P. Fenn, *Christian Higher Education in Changing China,
   1880–1950* (Grand Rapids, Mich.: William Eerdmans 1976), 203–8
75 R.C. Spooner, 'In West China,' *United Church Record and
   Missionary Review*, Nov. 1938
76 Ibid., also UCC-BFM-WCUU 12-4, L.G. Kilborn to J.H. Arnup and
   Armstrong, 7 June 1938
77 UCC-BFM-WCM 8-185, L.G. Kilborn to J.H. Arnup, 8 Jan. 1941, 3
78 UCC-BFM-WCM 9-223, L.G. Kilborn to J.H. Arnup, 13 Apr. 1943
79 Most of these came from National Central University and the

China Medical Board (PUMC). See, for example, RAC 1V2B9-159-1156, E.C. Forkner to Lobenstine, 15 Feb. 1945

80 UCC-BFM-WCUU 8-192, R.C. Spooner to Friends, 27 Jan. 1941, 3
81 UCC-BFM-WCM 90220, R.C. Spooner to J.H. Arnup, 24 Jan. 1943
82 *Ibid.*, 8-192, R.C. Spooner to J.H. Arnup, 29 June 1941, 3
83 This was the opinion of the Medical Education Committee of the American Board for China Christian Colleges. See UCC-BFM-BOM, box 30, Minutes of Subcommittee, 19 Apr. 1944, and Minutes of Meeting of Committee on Medical Education, 25 Sept. 1944
84 In 1944 Gerald Bell warned about the potential crisis in funding after the war ended. See UCC-BFM-WCM 10-238, Bell to J.H. Arnup, 31 Mar. 1944
85 RAC IV2B9 159-1156, C.E. Forkner to Lobenstine, 24 Jan. 1945
86 RAC IV2B9-159-1155, Chang to Balfour, 20 Sept. 1945
87 RAC IV2B9-158-1154, Minutes of China Medical Board, 31 May, 1945, no. 955
88 See UCC-BFM-WCM 11-264, Gladys Cunningham to J.H. Arnup, 8 Nov. 1946, and 11-270, Kilborn to Bell, 3 July 1946
89 Ibid.
90 UCC-BFM-WCM 11-270, L.G. Kilborn to Gerald Bell and J.H. Arnup, 3 Feb. 1946, and 12-295, L.G. Kilborn to J.H. Arnup, 12 July 1948
91 UCC-BFM-WCM 11-284, L.G. Kilborn to J.H. Arnup 19 Feb. 1947. Also 10-256, Kilborn to Arnup, 20 Aug. 1945, and 10-239, Kilborn to Gerald Bell, 17 Oct. 1944
92 Cunningham correspondence, Gladys Cunningham to family, 3 Jan. 1928
93 UCC-BFM-WCM 3-51, 'Report of Work,' 1929, A.E. Best
94 UCC-BFM-WCUU 1-13, L.G. Kilborn to J. Endicott, 7 Aug. 1931, 2
95 UCC-BFM-WCM 4-95, 'Annual Report of Work,' 1933, H.B. Collier, 5 Feb. 1934, 2
96 UCA personal papers, A.W. Lindsay, 'West China Union University,' 21 Mar. (1937?)
97 RAC RQ1 Ser. 601-21-193, C.C. Ch'en to Hume, 21 Mar. 1936
98 RAC RG1 Ser. 601-21-194, Grant (PUMC) to Gregg (CMB), 11 Nov. 1938
99 See, for example UCC-BFM-WCUU 12-3, J.H. Arnup to Cartwright (Methodist Episcopal Board, New York), 22 June 1938
100 UCC-BFM-WCM 7-160, Alice Lindsay to J.H. Arnup, 8 Oct. 1939
101 UCC-BFM-WCM 8-167, Ashley Lindsay to J.H. Arnup, 11 Aug. 1940, and 8-185, 11 Aug. 1941, 2

102 RAC IV2B9-159-1155, Lincoln Dsang, president of WCUU, to Board of Governors, WCUU, 20 Sept. 1943

103 Ibid., Lobenstine to J.H. Arnup, 10 Dec. 1943, 1

104 UCC-BFM-WCM 11-269, O. Joliffe to J.H. Arnup and Ballon, 21 Jan. 1946

105 UCC-BFM-WCM 11-284, L.G. Kilborn to J.H. Arnup, 30 Dec. 1947

106 UCC-BOM-WCM 13-331, Gladys Cunningham to J.H. Arnup, 7 Sept. 1950

107 UCC-BOM-WCM 13-341, J.H. Arnup, 6 Feb. 1951

108 UCC-BOM-WCM 13-339, Li Yuan, 'American Imperialist Missionaries in the Service of God,' *Chengdu Industrial and Commercial Guide Daily Paper*, 25 Nov. 1950

109 RAC RG4 Ser. 1-90-2108, Joseph Beech to Greene, 7 Feb. 1925, 2

110 UCC-BFM-WCUU 1-3, Registration with the Government, Oct. 1927

111 Ibid.

112 Ibid., and UCC-BFM-WCUU 1-3, Joseph Beech to Board of Governors, WCUU, 15 Feb. 1928

113 RAC IV2B9-124-902, Houghton to Greene, 8 Feb. 1927

114 UCA-WCUU pamphlets, 'West China Union University.' The University was also granted an absolute charter by the Regents of the University of the State of New York in 1934.

115 UCC-BFM-WCM 5-107, WCM 'Report of Work,' 1934

116 Ibid., 5-119, Dickinson to J. Endicott, 22 July 1935

117 UCC-BFM-WCUU 12-18, 'Twenty-five Years of Dentistry'

118 Interview with Mrs H.J. (Bea) Mullett

119 UCC-BFM-WCM 6-140, 'Report of Work,' 1927, T.H. Williams, 2

120 UCC-BFM-WCUU 9-230, 'WCUU Report,' 1943

121 DEA 19-CR-2-40, Dr E.S.W. Cheo, National Dental Health Board, to T.C. Davis, Canadian ambassador to China, 5 Jan. 1949

122 DEA 19-CR-24040, Embassy of the Republic of China, to Lester Pearson, secretary of state for external affairs, Ottawa, 11 Jan. 1949

123 Ibid., 2 Apr. 1949, attachment

124 Ibid., 24 July 1948, and 12 Mar. 1951

125 RAC RG1 Ser. 601-21-194, L.G. Kilborn to Grant, 26 Oct. 1938

126 Ibid., 18-161, 'First Report of the Szechuan Provincial Health Administration,' May–Dec. 1939, 1

127 Ibid., 'State and Local Health Services,' 1 Nov. 1940

128 Ibid., 18-162, 'Report of Public Health Training in Chengtu,' C.C. Chen, June 1944, 2

129 Interview with Dr C.C. Chen, Toronto, 5 Nov. 1979

130 UCC-BFM-WCM 8-175, Gerald Bell to J.H. Arnup, 9 July 1941
131 Ibid., 9-196, Gerald Bell to J.H. Arnup, 24 Feb. 1942
132 Interview with Dr Chen
133 UCA-UCC personal papers, Leslie Kilborn, 'Principles of Cooperation Between UNRRA and the Medical Missions' (no date); and DEA 6048-4c, L.G. Kilborn to Menzies, 23 Nov. 1944
134 UCC-BFM-BOM, box 30, Minutes of Meeting of Committee on Medical Education, ABCCC, 24 Mar. 1944, 2
135 Interview with Dr A.S. Allen, and documents on his imprisonment in UCC-BFM-WCM 14-359; DEA 3051-40, and Allen's personal correspondence
136 UCC-BFM-WCM 13-345, J.H. Arnup, 'China and Missions,' 24 Jan. 1951

Chapter 4

1 In 1944 the name was again changed to 'Board of Overseas Missions.' United Church of Canada Archives (UCA) references correspondingly change from BFM (Board of Foreign Missions) to BOM (Board of Overseas Missions) after 1944.
2 UCC-BFM-BOM (BWM), Joint Medical and Policy Committee, 1937–60, and UCC-BFM-WMS, Medical Board Minutes, 1927–47. This is contained in four volumes.
3 O.L. Kilborn, *Heal the Sick: An Appeal for Medical Missions in China* (Toronto: The Missionary Society of the Methodist Church 1910) 21
4 Valentin Rabe, 'Evangelical Logistics: Mission Support and Resources to 1920,' in J.K. Fairbank ed., *The Missionary Enterprise in China and America* (Cambridge, Mass.: Harvard University Press 1974), 71
5 Kilborn, *Heal the Sick*, 21–2
6 Ibid., 38–41
7 See John W. Foster, 'The Imperialism of Righteousness: Canadian Protestant Missions and the Chinese Revolution, 1925-1928,' (Ph.D. dissertation, University of Toronto 1977); chap. 1, n. 18.
8 Kilborn, *Heal the Sick*, 44
9 Wong Chimin and Wu Lien-teh, *History of Chinese Medicine* (Shanghai: National Quarantine Service 1936), 443, 464
10 W.R. Lambuth, *Medical Missions: The Twofold Task* (New York: Student Volunteer Movement 1920), preface
11 Ibid., Appendix A

12 Rabe, 'Evangelical Logistics,' 73–4
13 Lambuth, *Medical Missions*, preface
14 The May Fourth Movement was initiated by a student demonstration at Beijing University against the Treaty of Versailles in 1919. The specific grievances against Japanese imperialist influence in China developed into a more far-reaching nationalist cultural movement. For an analysis of the movement, see Chow Tse-tsung, *The May Fourth Movement* (Stanford: Stanford University Press 1960).
15 This movement was also primarily a student movement, directed against Christian missionaries in particular and foreigners in general. It was strongly influenced by communist organizers who identified the missionaries as 'the vanguards' of imperialist aggression. A concise analysis of this period can be found in T. Yamamoto and S. Yamamoto, 'The Anti-Christian Movement in China, 1922–1927,' *Far Eastern Quarterly* 12: 133–48 (February 1953).
16 An account of the incidents leading up to the evacuation, and the events following it, can be found in Stephen Endicott, *J.G. Endicott, Rebel out of China* (Toronto: University of Toronto Press 1980), chap. 9, 10. Archival references to the evacuation are found in UCC-BFM-WCM 1-5, 1926
17 UCA-WCUU pamphlet, 'Spend Ten Minutes in China,' 1919–20?, 16
18 UCC-BFM-WCM 1-18, 'Devolution,' 24 March 1927, 23, 2
19 UCA (uncatalogued in 1977), 'Report of the Special Committee on Policy (Medical Work),' 1936. (May be with E. Struthers, personal papers; one copy in writer's file.)
20 International Missionary Council, *The World Mission of the Church: Findings and Recommendations of the Meeting of the International Missionary Council; Tambaram, Madras, India, December 12–29, 1938* (London and New York: IMC 1939), 904, 99–100, 96–7. Among the representatives at this council meeting were Fong Su-hsuen, vice-chancellor of WCUU; Dr R.B. McClure, medical missionary from the United Church Mission in Honan, China; and K.C. Wong, MD, vice-president of the China Medical Association and secretary of the Commission on Medical Work of the National Christian Council of China.
21 UCA, 'Report of the Special Committee on Policy.'
22 'Free China' referred to that part of China that was not under Japanese military occupation. (See Wilder Penfield, 'Notes on a Brief Visit to Free China,' Appendix B, C922, National Research

Council of Canada.) Penfield's report has the following significance: 'This report, which was made available at the time to External Affairs and the armed forces, appears as an appendix to the October 1943 meeting of the Subcommittee on Surgery of NRC's Associate Committee on Medical Research. Dr Penfield was the chairman of this sub-committee and visited China as an extension of his visit to Russia for the purpose of improving wartime liaison on medical matters.' (Personal correspondence to the author from A.W. Tickner, Senior Archival Officer, National Research Council of Canada, 21 November 1978)

23 See chapter 3 of this book on the West China Union University, passim.

24 Wilder Penfield, 'China Mission Accomplished,' *Canadian Medical Association Journal* 26 August 1967, 468

25 UCA biographical files, 'Rev. Dr. C.W. Service,' 1898

26 UCA biographical files, 'Dr. W.J. Sheridan,' 1906. Subsequent data on application forms is from UCA biographical files.

27 UCA biographical files, 'Dr. W.G. Campbell,' 1936

28 Kilborn, *Heal the Sick*

29 See UCC-BFM-WMS, 'Medical Board Minutes,' 1940, regarding the appointment of a psychiatric consultant on the medical board.

30 The editor of an American missionary journal had suggested in 1918 that returning Christian soldiers 'should not be demobilized. They should simply be redistributed.' *Men and Missions* 10: 100 (December 1918), cited in Rabe, 'Evangelical Logistics,' 71

31 Clifton J. Phillips, 'The Student Volunteer Movement,' in Fairbank, *Missionary Enterprise*, 105, 100

32 Gilbert Reid, 1894, cited in Phillips, 'Student Volunteer,' 106

33 It was generally agreed that forty years was the maximum term of service, after which missionaries retired with a pension from the Board of Foreign Missions. UCA, biographical files, 'W.E. Smith'

34 UCA, personal papers, Leslie Kilborn.

35 M.C. Urquhart, ed., *Historical Statistics of Canada* (Cambridge: Cambridge University Press 1965), Series A 114–32, 18

36 While not statistically significant, it is noteworthy that five of the sixty were born in Asia, i.e., they were second-generation missionaries who returned to China as medical missionaries.

37 RAC-RG4 1-90-2109, Dr P.H. Stevenson, 'Report on West China Union University,' May 1926

38 A. Flexner, *Medical Education in the United States and Canada* (New York: Carnegie Foundation 1910), cited in H.E. MacDermot,

One Hundred Years of Medicine in Canada (Toronto: McClelland and Stewart 1967), 112. The information in the paragraph on medical education in Canada is based on MacDermot's book.

39 RAC-RG4, Stevenson, 'Report,' 8, 13
40 Lay ministers were not ordained by the church.
41 H.R. Isaacs, *Images of Asia (Scratches on our Minds)* (New York: Harper and Row 1972; originally published by MIT Press in 1958), 127–8
42 Of sixty medical missionaries, data on motivations are available for only forty. These are based on biographical files, personal correspondence, and interviews.
43 UCA biographical files, 'Dr I. Hilliard'
44 Ibid., 'Dr R. Hayward'
45 Interview with Dr A.S. Allen
46 UCA biographical files, 'Dr A.S. Allen'
47 UCA biographical files, pre-1921 application forms
48 UCA biographical files, 'Dr R. Outerbridge'
49 UCA biographical files, application forms
50 UCA biographical files, 'Eleanor Burwell'
51 UCA biographical files, 'Dr I. Hilliard'
52 Interview with Dr I. Hilliard, Toronto
53 UCA biographical files, 'Dr Outerbridge'
54 Interview with Dr Hilliard
55 UCA biographical files, 'Wolfendale,' 'Jones'
56 UCA biographical files, 'Wilford'
57 UCA biographical files, 'Dr Simpson'
58 UCA personal papers, A.W. Lindsay, file 2, 'Has the Church a Task Abroad?'
59 Personal correspondence, Dr R. Hayward, circular letter en route, 1933, no date or salutation, 2, 7
60 Personal correspondence, Dr E.R. Cunningham, en route to Chengdu, undated (1922–3)
61 O. Temkin, *The Double Face of Janus* (Baltimore: Johns Hopkins University Press 1977), 58
62 G. Rosen, 'The Hospital: Historical Sociology of a Community Institution,' in E. Freidson ed., *The Hospital in Modern Society*, (London: Collier-Macmillan 1963), 1–36
63 Temkin, *Double Face*, 49, and Rosen, 'The Hospital,' 23
64 Temkin, *Double Face*, 49
65 Harding Le Riche, 'Seventy Years of Public Health in Canada,' *Canadian Journal of Public Health* 70: 158 (May–June 1979)

66 S. Leff and V. Leff, *From Witchcraft to World Health* (New York: Macmillan 1958), chap. 1, and Temkin, *Double Face*, 437
67 Leff and Leff, *Witchcraft*
68 Personal communication; Dr J. Morrison; and H.E. MacDermot, *One Hundred Years*
69 MacDermot, *One Hundred Years*
70 D.W. Gullet, *A History of Dentistry in Canada* (Toronto: University of Toronto Press 1971). The information on the dental profession is based on this source.
71 See B.R. Blishen, *Doctors and Doctrines: The Ideology of Medical Care in Canada* (Toronto: University of Toronto Press 1969).
72 Johnson, *Professions and Power* (London: Macmillan 1972, 81
73 Phillips, 'Student Volunteer Movement,' 104
74 Fairbank, *Missionary Enterprise*, 7

Chapter 5

1 These estimates were repeated in numerous anecdotal reports from a variety of sources. There is no documented evidence available.
2 The original number of names on the list was 128, but two were deceased.
3 Of the questionnaire respondents, 15 of 36 (42 per cent) were 1930s graduates; 26 of 91 (29 per cent) were 1940s graduates.
4 West China University of Medical Sciences (WCUMS) Archives, file 12, document 10
5 United Church of Canada Archives (UCA)-UCC-BFM-WCUU II:59, 'Place of Origin of WCUU Students.'
6 UCA-WCUU pamphlet, 'The West China Union University, 1910-1939,' 22
7 WCUMS file 12, doc. 10, 'Student Records,' 1937–8
8 These rates drop dramatically for the few families who reported having a fourth child. Only 50 per cent of these children attended university, likely because their adolescence coincided with the Cultural Revolution.
9 Jessie Lutz agrees that the Christian college middle schools served as 'feeder' schools to the universities. She notes that the emphasis on science laboratory work and English in the Christian schools gave their students a competitive edge over government school graduates. (Personal communication to the author, May 1991.) See later reference to Lutz.
10 UCA-UCC-BFM-WCUU II:59, 'Christian Students,' Spring 1946

11 WCUMS file 12, doc. 12. This document indicates that Christian students came from poorer families than non-Christian students.

12 The following section is based on an interview with one of the alumni in Chengdu, and corroborated by survey data.

13 One anecdotal report suggested that students at National Central University were more likely to read *bai hua* (colloquial Chinese) novels than foreign literature. The WCUU students felt that they were beyond the limitations of feudal family constraints, which was the theme of many *bai hua* novels, and thus were more open to Western influence than their less sophisticated peers.

14 WCUMS file 12, doc. 8b, 'Class of 1943 Student Records'

15 Thirty-two of these applications were reviewed in detail. WCUMS file 12, doc. 11

16 Ibid.

17 Cited in Peter Mitchell, 'Women and the Healing Profession,' draft, 1991, 5. WCUU was one of the last of the Christian universities to admit women. Jessie G. Lutz, *China and the Christian Colleges, 1850–1950* (Ithaca and London: Cornell University Press 1971), 136

18 UCC-BFM-WCUU 1-2, Beech to Flavelle, 23 Nov. 1926

19 The Wanxian incident in 1926 was one of a series of clashes between British and Japanese imperialists, and Chinese student- and worker-led nationalistic protests against Western domination of China. In this particular incident, British and Japanese gunboats fired on the Sichuanese city of Wanxian, on the Yangzi River. The event which triggered this chain of events was the May 30th Incident in 1925, in which 3000 students marched in Nanjing to protest British and Japanese killings of Chinese workers and students during various strikes and demonstrations. British police in Nanjing opened fire on the demonstrators, killing eleven students, wounding many others, and arresting the student leaders.

20 UCC-BFM-WCM 1-5, Sparling *'Re Agitation in the WCUU,'* 4–8 Oct. 1926, and RAC RGIV2B9-124-900, Yard to Vincent, 7 Jan. 1927

21 Cunningham Correspondence, Gladys Cunningham to family, 9 May 1926

22 Ibid. E.R. Cunningham to Ted, 19 Aug. 1926

23 Ibid.

24 UCC-BFM-WCM 3-66, 'Report of the UCC-WCM,' 1931, L.G. Kilborn, 14

25 UCC-BFM-WCM 5-121, 'WCM Report of Work for the year,' 1935

26 UCC-BFM-WCM 4-95, 'Annual Report of Work: 1933,' B. Collier, 5 Feb. 1934

27 Confidential source; corroborated by interview with William Small, Toronto, 26 Oct. 1981

28 Interview with Dr W.G. Campbell, Winnipeg. This view is widely held by alumni in Chengdu.

29 WCUMS file 12

30 For an account of campus politics during the war, see Hu Kuo-tai, 'The Struggle between the Kuomintang and the Chinese Communist Party on Campus during the War of Resistance, 1937–45,' China Quarterly 118: 300–23 (June 1988)

31 Huaxi Xiehe Daxue Xiaokan (no date, between 1937 and 1949)

32 L.G. Kilborn, personal papers, note from E.R. Cunningham (no date)

33 Mary Brown Bullock, An American Transplant: The Rockefeller Foundation and Peking Union Medical College (Berkeley: University of California Press 1981)

34 Phillip West, Yenching University and Sino-Western Relations, 1916–1952 (Cambridge, Mass.: Harvard University Press 1976)

35 Lutz, China

36 Bullock, American Transplant, 109, 112, 113

37 See Y.C. Wang, Chinese Intellectuals and the West, 1872–1949 (Chapel Hill: University of North Carolina Press 1966), 13; and Marie Claude Bergere, 'The Role of the Bourgeoisie,' in M.C. Wright, ed., China in Revolution: The First Phase, 1900–1913, (New Haven and London: Yale University Press 1968), 229–95

38 Bullock, American Transplant, 128–9

39 Philip West, Yenching University and Sino-Western Relations, 1916–1952 (Cambridge, Mass.: Harvard University Press 1976), 138, 139, 279, 142

40 Lutz, China 71, 76

41 Ibid., 166, 304, 309

42 Ibid., 342, 73

43 Ibid., 372

44 RAC IV2B9-158-1154, United Board for Christian Colleges in China, 'Preliminary Data on Mission Medical Schools in China,' 15 June 1954

45 UCC-BFM-WCM 1-13, Kilborn to Endicott, 7 Aug. 1931, 2

46 UCC-BFM-WCM 'Report of Work for 1934,' 7

47 UCC-BFM-WCM 3-66, 'Report,' 1931, L.G. Kilborn

48 UCA-WCUU pamphlets, 'The West China Union University, 1910–1939,' 24

49 UCC-BFM-WCM 5-111, Bell to Endicott, 26 June 1935, 4

50 UCC-BFM-WCUU, box 30, American Board of China Christian Colleges, Committee on Medical Education, 24 Mar. 1944, Appendix A
51 DEA 6048-40C, R. McClure to Wilder Penfield re: Condition of Chinese Military Medical Services, 27 Sept. 1943, 2
52 American Board; and McClure to Penfield

Chapter 6

1 This statement was attributed to Dr Ed Cunningham. Personal communication from alumni to the author
2 Leslie G. Kilborn, 'Our Last Term in China: 1949–52.' Unpublished account, in the United Church Archives, Toronto, UCC-BFM-WCM 14-36
3 Vice-President Guo Mo-ruo, speech at the 65th meeting of the State Administrative Council, 29 Dec., 1950, in Kilborn, 'Our Last Term,' 7
4 WCUU Archives, Chengdu, file 221. The term *wei* was used to denote any organizations or institutions which existed under the Guomindang regime and were therefore regarded as illegitimate in the new Communist regime. It has been translated as 'enemy,' 'false,' and 'so-called.'
5 Ibid., *Huaxi Xiehe Daxue Xiaokan*, 3 June 1949
6 Zhang Lin-gao died in prison. His name was officially rehabilitated in a posthumous ceremony in 1989. This is a Chinese Communist ritual whereby those accused of political wrongdoings in the past are exonerated and their good name 'restored.'
7 This was reported in Kilborn's, 'Our Last Term,' and corroborated by numerous interviews with alumni.
8 Those who became Communist Party members reportedly had more influence than those who did not. Personal communication to the author
9 Of four other respondents who indicated that they narrowly escaped being labelled as Rightists, two were also woman graduates of the 1930s. One can only speculate that these women, whose retirement age in China is earlier than men by five years, were more dispensable than their male colleagues. They may also have been in less senior positions.
10 There are numerous accounts of the experiences of intellectuals during the Cultural Revolution. See Anne F.Thurston, *Enemies of the People* (Cambridge, Mass.: Harvard University Press 1988).

188 Notes to pages 137–49

11 Zhou Beilong and Huang Shiqi, 'The Prospects of Education in China Towards the Year 2000,' in Lo Fu-chen, ed., *Asian and Pacific Economy Towards the Year 2000* (Kuala Lumpur: Asian and Pacific Development Centre 1987), 343–4
12 Ibid., 329
13 It is likely that medicine includes dentistry in these statistics, since dentistry is considered a branch of medicine, known as stomatology, and the duration of training is roughly the same.
14 Department of Planning, Ministry of Education, People's Republic of China. *Achievement of Education in China: Statistics, 1949–1983* (Beijing: People's Publishing House 1985), 108, 114, 102–3, 105
15 For example, a stamp commemorating Zhu Ke-zhen (1890–1974), a Western-trained meteorologist; Wu You-Xun (1897–1977), a physicist; and Hua Luo-gen, China's premier mathematician, who died in 1985.
16 *People's Daily*, 27 Aug. 1987
17 *China Daily*, 1 Feb. 1989, 5. See also C.C. Chen, *Medicine in Rural China: A Personal Account* (Berkeley: University of California Press 1989).
18 Dean T. Jamison, et al., *China: The Health Sector* (Washington, DC: World Bank, 1984)
19 Ibid., 102–5
20 It is not known when each respondent joined the Communist Party, but it is assumed that only a small minority (who were identified by their peers) joined before the late 1970s. Personal communications to the author

Chapter 7

1 This quote is taken from an American study of the secularization of foreign aid: Edwin Bock, *Fifty Years of Technical Assistance* (Chicago: Public Administration Clearing House 1954), 2.
2 Interview with Dr George C. A. Deng. West China University of Medical Sciences, Chengdu, Sichuan, Oct. 1986
3 For a recent discussion of this issue see OECD, *Twenty-Five years of Development Cooperation: 1985 Report*, (Paris: OECD 1985), 278
4 Richard Allen, *The Social Passion: Religion and Social Reform in Canada, 1914–28* (Toronto: University of Toronto Press 1973), 3
5 UCA-MCC-MEM-WCM 2-36, Sutherland to Kilborn, 31 Aug. 1908
6 Correspondence and personal documents of Dr Gladys Cunning-

ham and numerous other missionary accounts of the time

7 Omar Kilborn, *Heal the Sick* (Toronto: Missionary Society of the Methodist Church 1910), 270

8 K.W. Thompson, *Foreign Assistance: A View from the Private Sector* (Notre Dame: University of Notre Dame Press 1972), 114

9 Indeed, contemporary foreign aid programs have begun to take into account the necessity of having the recipient society participate in the design and delivery of technology transfer and education.

10 Thomas Metzger, *Escape from Predicament: Neoconfucianism and China's Evolving Political Culture* (New York: Columbia Univesity Press 1977), 194, 196

11 I am grateful to Jerome Chen for his comments, early in the development of this study, on the relevance of the socialization of this cohort.

12 Merle Goldman et al., *China's Intellectuals: Advise and Dissent* (Cambridge, Mass.: Harvard University Press 1981); T. Cheek and C. Hamrin, *China's Establishment Intellectuals* (Armonk, NY: M.E. Sharpe 1986); Li Zehou and Vera Schwarcz, 'Six Generations of Modern Chinese Intellectuals,' *Chinese Studies in History* 17: 42–56 (Winter 1983–4); Vera Schwarcz, 'Behind a Partially-Open Door: Chinese Intellectuals and the Post-Mao Reform Process,' *Pacific Affairs* 59: 577–604 (1986); Merle Goldman and Denis Simon, 'The Onset of China's New Technological Revolution,' in Denis Simon and Merle Goldman, eds., *Science and Technology in Post-Mao China* (Cambridge, Mass.: Harvard University Press 1989)

13 Li Zehou and Schwarcz, 'Six Generations'

14 The six groups are (1) the feudal intellectuals of the 1898 Reform movement; (2) the May Fourth intellectuals who experienced the failure of the 1911 Revolution; (3) the 'enlightenment' intellectuals of the 1920s; (4) the Anti-Japanese War generation of the 'turbulent 1930s and wartime 1940s; (5) the 'liberation' generation of the contented 1950s; and (6) the 'troublesome' Red Guard generation. They comment that the seventies were 'bleak,' and that the 1980s intellectuals experienced an awakening after decades of political repression.

15 Julian Marias, *Generations: A Historical Method*, trans. by Harold C. Raley (Alabama: University of Alabama Press 1970)

16 Vera Schwarcz, 'Behind a Partially Open Door' 589

17 Ibid., 590

18 Cheek and Hamrin, *China's Establishment Intellectuals*

19 Michel Bonnin and Yves Chevrier, 'The Intellectual and the State:

Social Dynamics of Intellectual Autonomy during the Post-Mao Era,' *China Quarterly*, 127: 572 (Sept. 1991)
20 Ibid., 593
21 David Apter, *The Politics of Modernization* (Chicago: University of Chicago Press 1965), chap. 5
22 Richard P. Suttmeier, 'Science, Technology, and China's Future – A Framework for Analysis,' in Denis Simon and Merle Goldman, eds., *Science and Technology in Post-Mao China*, 395–6

Index

Africa, 17, 53
Allen, A. Stewart, 34, 74, 80
alumni (WCUU), 11–12, 18, 35, 38, 59, 61, 67–8, 76, 106–8, 124–46, 150–2, 156–7; associations of WCUU, 107, 144–5, 154; of Christian colleges, 20, 118; generations of, 9–10, 25, 108, 110–12, 118, 124–45, 152–3, 156 (*see also* generations); medical and dental, 121–3; networks, 144–5, 154; 1960s generation of alumni, 142; surviving, 136
American. *See* foreigners
anatomy, 93
anti-Christian movement, 36–7, 43, 66–7, 80, 86, 114, 117
anti-elitism. *See* elites
anti-intellectual. *See* elites, intellectuals
Anti-Rightist Campaign, 20, 133
Apter, David, 20–1, 24, 154
archives, 11, 108, 110; Department of External Affairs (Canada), 7; Rockefeller Foundation China Medical Board (RAC-CMB), 7, 91; United Church of Canada (UCA),

7, 108; West China University of Medical Sciences (WCUMS), 8, 108, 110, 128. *See also* methodology
Association of American Medical Colleges, 55
Austria, 93

Bai, Yingcai, 69
Band, William, 54
Banting, Frederick, 93
bao jia system. *See* Chinese society
barefoot doctors, 135
Barotseland, 17
Barter, A.J., 34
Beech, Joseph, 45, 62, 70–1
Beh, Y.T. *See* Bai, Yingcai
Beijing, 10, 18, 26, 47, 113, 131, 136, 141, 144
Bell, Gerald, 63
Best, Charles, 93
Bethune, Norman, 14
Bismarck, 100
Board of Foreign Missions, 66, 77, 80, 82–4
Borodin, 14
Borthwick, Sally, 22

117, 123, 148, 152. *See also*
Chinese society
corruption, 41
Crawford, W., 72
Cultural Revolution, 7, 11, 23,
133–4, 136, 142, 144
Cunningham, Ed R., 32, 115
Cunningham, Gladys, 59, 66, 69,
114

Dalhousie University, 92
Daoist Temples, 151
Deng, Xiaoping, 24, 139
Deng, Xi-hou, 40, 128
dentistry, 54, 60, 132; alumni, 132;
College of Dentistry, 60, 62–3,
71–2, 98; education, 55–6, 59;
faculty of, 132; modern, 132;
profession, 102; students, 110,
116. *See also* alumni; A.W.
Lindsay; H.J. Mullett; National
Dental Board of Health; Dr
Thompson; West China Dental
Association; West China Union
University, College of Medicine
and Dentistry
devolution, 57, 61–2, 66–70, 74–5,
80, 82, 121
Dingxian, 139
Dsang, Lincoln. *See* Zhang, Lin-gao

East China, 57–8, 108, 114, 121
education, 138, 142
– Christian, 44, 65, 144, 149;
universities, 5, 8, 18–19, 45–6,
53, 55, 60, 118–21. *See also*
alumni; United Board for
Christian Colleges in China
– dental, *see* dentistry
– destruction of educational
system, 137

– girls', 113
– government, 68–9, 110, 115,
118–20; municipal health
workers school, 129
– higher, *see* university
– medical, 4, 47, 50, 53, 57, 59,
60–2, 69, 71, 74, 76, 78, 82, 93,
119, 121, 125, 126, 131–3, 141,
143, 153; medical schools, 132–3,
138; military medical school,
129; research institutes, 131;
research-oriented schools, 147;
Western model of, 155
– middle school, 110
– missionary, 5, 19, 43, 68, 110,
112, 115, 119, 133
– models of, 45, 126, 155; foreign,
125, 155; Soviet, 131, 140
– modern, 118
– pharmacy, *see* West China
Union University
– policy, 140; academic ranks, 137.
See also science
– political, 18, 130
– post-graduate 137–8, 141, 143
– primary, 110
– reform, 140
– religious, 111
– research and teaching, 144
– science, 13, 15, 25, 44, 46, 54–5,
77, 80–1, 87, 113, 115, 120, 124,
131, 150, 153; basic, 143; basic
sciences and research, 142
– specialized schools and research
institutes, 154
– standards, 142
– technology, 13, 17, 23, 46, 54,
87, 104, 125, 151
– traditional Chinese, 120
– university, 3, 9–10, 24, 64–5, 70,
109, 114–15, 119–20, 125–7, 133,